AN EIGHT-HUNDRED YEAR OLD BOOK OF INDIAN MEDICINE AND FORMULAS

AN EIGHT-HUNDRED YEAR OLD BOOK OF INDIAN MEDICINE AND FORMULAS

TRANSLATED FROM THE ORIGINAL VERY OLD HINDI INTO GUJARATI CHARACTER AND THENCE INTO ENGLISH

BY

ELIZABETH SHARPE

GYAN

Published by

GYAN

Gyan Publishing House
5, Ansari Road
Daryaganj, New Delhi-110002
Phone: 011-47034999, 9811692060
E-mail: books@gyanbooks.com

Distribution Network
gyanbooks.com
India, USA, Canada, UK, Australia, France

ISBN : 978-81-212-4517-3 (HB)
First Published, London, 1937

2nd Impression 2020

Printed at: Gyan Press, Delhi.

An Eight-Hundred Year Old Book of Indian Medicine and Formulas
Author: Elizabeth Sharpe

DEDICATION

TO

HIS HIGHNESS MAHARANA SHRI SIR DAULAT SINHJI,

K.C.I.E., K.C.S.I.,

Thakore Sahib of Limbdi,

Whose love of scholarship has made the translation of many old manuscripts of India possible.

TRANSLATOR'S NOTE

The translator is a complete lay-woman where medicine is concerned. Latin and English names owe their origin to the Court physician; but many others, where uncertainty occurs, have, necessarily, to be left in their vernacular form.

The book, despite its incomplete form, has taken the best part of four years; later, she was ill; and Vaid-Raj Gunadhya Amritlal Pattani, the Limbdi Court physician, who worked tirelessly for her giving her the equivalents both in Latin and English, died when the work was still unfinished.

It has, therefore, to go to the press in its present incomplete state; but even in this state, it may well prove a valuable contribution to those rare manuscripts already translated: for it is the writer's own copy; the only one in existence.

This manuscript is very tender, and it is possible it may not last many years longer.

The original is in a peculiar form of Hindi. The original verses are in couplets; they show unusual talent and make pleasing melody.

The writer was the pupil of the great Jain priest Hemchand, who founded the "gadi" of the non-idol worshipping sect of the Jains:[1] and was himself therefore a monk.

Many of these medicines, especially the ointments, used with our modern antiseptics appear worth a trial.

Mear House,
Kempsey, Worcester.

Oct. 21*st*, 1936.

[1] *See* the translator's biography of the Thakore Sahib of Limbdi (John Murray), pp. 109-110.

CONTENTS

PART I

CONTENTS

CONTENTS

PART II

PART III

PART IV

PART V

Powders

CONTENTS

PART VI

PILLS

PART VII

OINTMENTS

CONTENTS

PART VIII

Oils

[Acknowledgments are due to Mr. Labhshankar of the Sir Jaswantsinhji High School for his invaluable scholarly help.]

AN EIGHT-HUNDRED YEAR OLD BOOK OF INDIAN MEDICINE AND FORMULAS

Translated by

ELIZABETH SHARPE, F.R.G.S., Etc.

(In the original, this is the last page of the manuscript.)

A Physician is much honoured amongst Kings and people ; he obtains desired objects ; he gets a palanquin, an honourable seat and good things to eat.

Many men and women stand at his door from sunrise.

All serve the physician and give him great honour ; indeed, the house of the physician is as great as that of a king.

Having known the greatness of a physician, the science of medicine has been studied and composed in " Dodhak "[1] metre.

I bow to the wise and beg their pardon if any defects remain.

The wise should study the verses, and look on them with a favourable eye rather than with the look of a cavilling critic. Waghji Muni, the disciple of Hemchandra makes this request.

These verses were composed in Samvat[2] 1491 of the second of Magh, Friday in the Rohini Nakshetra.

Jeychand Sur was born 5th in the line of the Gaucha (clan) of Pashchand whose members are famous all over the world.

Shri Vraddhchand was the store-house of all merits and head of them all.

His disciple was Hemchandra, very learned and famous amongst all learned men.

His disciple of small talent composed these verses.

Waghji Muni.

[1] " Dodhak "—Couplets. [2] 1435 A.D. In the month of February.

NOTE

The first page of the manuscript is missing.

All words in brackets are the original Hindi ones. Where there was the slightest doubt, the original word in Hindi has been left.

I

DELIRIUM—BHAGNA NETRA

The remedies are as follows :—

1. Syrapus rotundas (daru-moth), trichosanthe cucumerina (patol-katu), a combination of terminalia bellerica, myrobalans and hogplums (trifala), solanum xanthocarpum (kshundra), turmeric and Indian lilace-tree fruit ; all these should be boiled together ; they will make a good medicine for curing delirium.

2. Mustard, dry ginger, peppera-longa and ordinary pepper (vyokh) pounded together in equal proportion with honey, asafœtida, sweet-flag root (vaj) make an excellent medicine for delirium.

3. Dry ginger, peppera-longa and ordinary pepper, winter cherries (asandh), cloves, salt, sweet-flag root, honey and garlic all pounded together and thrown in the urine of a she-goat make a good medicine for delirium.

4. Synapis alba (asarasav), spykenard valeriana (tagar), cotton seeds, costus root (kuth), cinnamon, cedar (devdar) and the root of gigantic solvert (arka) should be pounded together with ghee (clarified butter).

That delirium (sunnipat) in which the eyes of the patient become blood-red and the patient's vision is impaired, is generally considered as incurable.

II

REMEDY FOR

PROFUSE MENSTRUATION—RAKTASRAVA

1. Berberis aristata (nisha-katu), fumigatory, fogonia arabica (dhanvavasak) and chiretta should be boiled together and eaten daily with sugar.

III

DELIRIUM—SUNNIPAT

In which the patient raves in an unconscious state.

1. Eaglewood (tagar), winter cherries, poparlind fig-tree (piparo), conscura decussata (funidadi), cedar (devdar), Indian plimywort (brahmi), pudding pipe tree (girmalo), cryapus rotundas (moth), Christmas rose (katuk), myrobalans (abhaya) and grapes together cure this delirium within 14 days.

IV

DISEASES OF THE TONGUE—JIBHAK

Characteristics and Symptoms

1. The tongue becomes hard.

2. There is weakness, deafness, stammering, hard breathing and cough ; there is uneasiness of the body : these are the symptoms of tongue diseases.

Cures for the Same

1. Glycyrrhiza glabra (madhurmuli, brinjal-seeds, dry ginger, Christmas rose (katuk), asafœtida, cyrapus rotundas (moth), clerodendron serrotum (bharangi), tinospora cordifolia (galo), pistacia integerrima (kaksingi), sweet-flag root, a prickly plant named hedy surum alhagi (dham-

aso), curcuma zedooria (sadhi), Indian plimywort (brahmi) should be boiled together, and then pounded together with cold water.

2. Cedar, pudding pipe tree, chiretta, orris root (pushkarmul), myrobalans, solanum xanthocarpum (kshundra), cyrapus rotundas (nagar moth) and . . . (harshul) should be crushed and pounded with the juice of the cytrus (bijora).

3. Dry ginger, white and black pepper should be smeared on the tongue.

V

DELIRIUM—TRIDOSH

Its Symptoms

There is sweetness in the mouth; the person is much inclined to sleep and sleeps long; there is uneasiness. The patient cannot breathe freely, cannot speak, perspires. These are the signs of this kind of delirium (tridosh).

Cures

1. Powdered asafœtida and dry ginger rubbed on the body cure this kind of delirium.

2. Garlic, pepper, sweet-flag root, salt, nitrate of potash, the seeds of butea frondosa (khakhra) pounded together in the urine of a cow cures this delirium.

3. The turbeeth root (shayman), a combination of ten roots (dashmula), clerodendron serratum (bharangi), orris root (pushkarmul), dill seeds, adhatoda vasica (vasa), curcuma zedooria (sadhi), tinospora cordifolia (galo) should be taken in equal proportions, boiled together and drunk.

4. Lemon, cyclea peltata (padhi), curcuma zedooria (sadhi) pepper, the roots of castor plant seeds, Bengal maderroots (majith), solanum xanthocarpum (kshundra),

plumbago zeylanica (chitrak), bell-tree root (biljada), salt, dry ginger, root of trianthema monogyne (vasith), turbeeth root (shayman), chiretta, hornbeam leaved cedar (bal) all taken in equal proportion cure this kind of delirium immediately.

VI

DYSENTERY—ATISAR

Dysentery is of three kinds due to excess of Wind (Vata); Bile (Pita); and Phlegm (Kafa). That in which there is acute pain and the patient feels lassitude is Wind (Vata) Dysentery (Atisar).

Cures

1. Desmodium gangeticum (salavan), vraria picta (pidhavani), padellium muracus (gokhru), wild brinjal seeds, kuskus grass (valo), dry ginger (nagar) should be crushed together; and the powder of these and citrus (amalvetsa), Indian mello (bal) and essence of pomegranate should be taken with fruit. This cures the Wind (Vata) dysentery.

2. Take half a "tank"[1] each of dry ginger, cyrapus rotundas (moth), kuskus grass (valo), bell-tree fruit powder (bilichur), fumigatory, flour of fried gram boiled together with simploces racemosa (lod), a sensitive plant named "lajalu," curcuma zedooria (padhi), dry ginger, coriander seeds, cyrapus rotundas (moth), tinospara cordifolia (giloi), bell-tree leaves and greaslia tomentosa (dhavdi). The boiled water should be drunk.

Bile (Pit) Dysentery

1. Bile dysentery is that in which there is blood in the fecal matter and the fecal matter has a very bad smell; there is burning sensation and fever.

[1] *See* Appendix B—Weights.

Cures

1. Sugar, dry ginger, costus root (kuthvadi), bell-tree fruit, cumin seeds and the water in which rice is boiled taken together cure this disease completely.

2. Akonatum atis (ativakh), bell-tree fruit, sweet-flag root, Christmas rose (kātuk) and cyrapus rotundas (moth) should be boiled together and dry ginger and akonatum atis (ativakh) should be taken with the water in which rice is boiled.

3. The gum of the red silk cotton tree, greaslia tomentosa (dhavdi), dry ginger, parsnip (ajmo) in equal quantities taken in whey made from cow's milk cures fever due to dysentery.

4. The gum of the red silk cotton tree (mochrasa), simploces racemosa (lod), greaslia tomentosa (dhavdi), oval-leaved rajabe (indrajava), bell-tree fruit juice (bilisar) boiled together and drunk cure dysentery.

5. Dry ginger, myrobalans (abhaya), cyrapus rotundas (moth), sweet-flag root (vaj), akonatum atis (ativakh) and cedar (devdar) boiled together and drunk cure this disease.

6. Padellium muracus (gokhru), oval-leaved rajabe (indrajava), the roots of the castor plant (arand) should be pounded together and taken with honey to cure dysentery.

7. Mesna ferrea (nagkeshar) of four kinds, pepper root (granthik), dry ginger, parsnip, coriander seeds, dill seeds, pepper, oval-leaved rajabe (indrajava), bilvoben, costus root (kuth), bell-tree fruit (bil), greaslia tomentosa (dhavdi), feronia elephantum (kauth), the bark of pomegranate and plumbago zeylanica (chitrak) all pounded together in equal proportion and taken cure dysentery.

8. Pepper root (granthik), sweet-flag root (vaj), plumbago zeylanica (chitrak) pounded together and taken as a medicine undoubtedly cure dysentery very quickly.

9. Resin (ral), sugar, taken with honey prevent dysentery (atisara), guavas, seeds of mango-tree, costus root, simploces racemosa (lod), bell-tree fruit, sweet-flag root, barley, licorice, cytrus, cyrapus rotundas (moth), dry ginger, kuskus grass (lochan), honey, greaslia tomentosa (dhavdi), pounded together and mixed with clarified butter (ghee) make a powder known as Gangadhar powder (churna) which cures dysentery; and the pill made of dry ginger and opium also gives happiness by curing this disease.

VII

HICCOUGH

1. If a man drinks licorice and pepper in a solution of sugar and then drink the juice of ocymum sanctum (tulshi) immediately afterwards his hiccough stops at once.

2. Dry ginger should be drunk with molasses, and the bark of the babul tree and the mango-tree should be boiled together and drunk; this will cure the hiccough at once.

3. Honey, licorice, and dry ginger pounded together with chiretta and drunk in water will cure this disease immediately.

VIII

COLD

1. Seeds of lotus, 30 cardemons, roasted paddy-seeds (lazakhan), pepper and cloves drunk with honey will remove cold.

2. Two leaves of pepper should be crushed with seven "pishang." A pill made of these of the size of a berry and eaten removes cold.

3. Having mixed Indian mello (kangsa) in the water,

which is being heated by repeatedly putting in heated gold, and drinking it after filtering, removes cold.

4. Dry ginger, coriander seeds, sandalwood, rose-cardemons and camphor should be boiled together, and drunk in the morning for removing cold.

5. Dry ginger, mineral salt, black and white pepper and cedar should be taken in small quantities with honey all in equal proportion to cure cold.

6. Myrobalans (harade), terminalia bellerica (beda), hogplums, dry ginger, bay breng (vavading) should be boiled together, and drunk with honey. This remedy will surely remove the cold.

7. Having boiled together according to the process of making medicines, peacock feathers with licorice, cloves, cardemons, tin, and pepper, it should be eaten with honey. This cures cold.

IX

THE ITCH—ECZEMA

1. Myrobalans, mineral salt (sindha), asculint flacursia . . . four lines ineligible owing to holes due to tenderness of the manuscript . . .

2. Mercury (ras), sulphur (ganthak), asculint flacursia (bavachi), oil of synapis alba (katuk oil) and yellow orpiment (harital) should be heated and applied to the body; this medicine will cure itch immediately.

3. Turmeric, blue vitriol, asculint flacursia (bavachi), carbonate of soda and sulphur should be mixed with double their quantity of "kupavadi" and rubbed on the body in the oil of synapis alba (katuk oil).

4. Sulphur and mercury should be powdered in oil and blue vitriol and cedar (devdar) mixed with them. If this oil is applied to the body, the itch will disappear.

X

BABHUTI

1. Lac (lakh), sodium carbonate, asculint flacursia (bavachi), salt, sulphur (amalsar) and fermented corn (kaji) applied cure "babhuti."

2. Seeds of radishes, turmeric, asculint flacursia (bavachi), cassia tora (puvad) and fermented corn (kaji) remove "babhuti" of the body.

XI

CURE FOR

HYDROCELE—ANTARGAL

1. To pierce the middle vein of the ear is the best way of curing hydrocele.

2. Heat should be given with "hastpandu" and "chanjap" and the last finger should be pierced . . . five lines omitted here . . . ineligible owing to tenderness of manuscript . . .

XII

JAUNDICE—KAMALA

1. Five "tanks"[1] of the juice of the Indian lilace tree (nimb tree) mixed with nine tanks of sugar should be drunk every morning for five days. It cures jaundice.

2. Cyrapus rotundas (moth), Christmas rose (katuk), berberis aristata (darunisha), horse radish tree (saradhu), costus root (kuth), cedar, pepper root, pistachia integerrima (singi), fumigatory, bamboo, chiretta, the bark of the Indian lilace tree (nimb tree), fenel seeds (shauff), and myrobalans, terminalia bellerica (beda) and hogplums should be boiled together and drunk for removing jaundice.

[1] *See* Appendix B—Weights

3. Turmeric, iron of myrobalans powdered and mixed with clarified butter (ghee) and honey and myrobalans mixed with treacle and honey cure jaundice.

4. Dry ginger, long pepper and black pepper (vyokh), turmeric, hogplums . . . one word worn out in the manuscript . . . honey, iron, mixed together cure jaundice.

5. A combination of dry ginger, long pepper and black pepper (trikatu), myrobalans, terminalia bellerica (beda) and hogplums, chiretta, adhatoda vasica (vasa), tinospara cordifolia (galo) of the Indian lilace tree should be boiled together, and the water drunk with honey. It is sure to cure jaundice.

XIII

COLIC—SHOOL

1. One "pala"[1] juice of citrus medica (bijora) with black pepper, soda bicarbonate, pepper root, sandalwood and clarified butter (ghee) cure the disease of colic.

XIV

CURE FOR POISONS

1. The pain of poison through eating the flesh of a wild boar is removed by drinking in whey pounded senna (sonamukhi), turbeeth root (nasotar) and the purgative nut plant.

2. Poison leaves the body altogether by taking myrobalans, terminalia bellerica, hogplums, nuxvomica (jherkochla), pepper, clarified butter, aconitum (vachhnag), and juice of brinjal as an emetic.

3. The poison of arsenic (somal) is removed by eating sweet pumpkin and pulp of benicassa cerifera (gir); and

[1] *See* Appendix B—Weights.

that of opium is removed by drinking randia dumeturum (mainal) paste rubbed on a stone with water.

4. Gassypium arboreum (hirdhan), coriander seeds, clarified butter, milk, curd, the urine and dung of a cow when drunk remove the poison of the thorn apple (dhatura), while the poison due to the juice of the ark (ankdo) is cured by applying myrobalan paste rubbed on a stone with water.

5. The poison of marking nuts (bhilama) is cured by eating gram fried in sesamum oil; and the poison from blue vitriol is cured by eating flour of wheat cooked in sugar (lapsi) or molasses, sugar or almonds.

XV

MEDICINE FOR

DYEING THE HAIR

1. Powder of iron should be placed in an iron vessel and the vessel should be heated on the fire. After an interval of an hour-and-a-half the vessel should be taken down from the fire; and the powder in it pounded in a mortar with a pestle, put back in the vessel, and the vessel again put on the fire. This process should continue for twelve hours.

Then the powder should be taken out of the vessel and mixed with ten "tanks"[1] of whey. It should then be put under the ground and heated thus for nine days; it should be taken out on the tenth day and pills made of it with alum (turi) and then in the morning this hair-dye should be applied and washed out with the juice of hogplums.

2. The seeds of feronia elephantum (kauth) with leaves, the roots of buchanania latifolia (piuki), flowers of pandonus adoratissimus (kevda) and troiling eclipta (bhangro) should be brought and left on the ground to be dried. When

[1] *See* Appendix B—Weights.

they are dried up, they should be put with myrobalans, terminalia bellerica and hogplums and oil of sesamum in an iron vessel under earth for one month. An ointment or dye for the hair will be ready which will make white hair black.

XVI

PAIN IN THE STOMACH

1. Turmeric, turbeeth root (nasotar), myrobalans (harade), groton triglium (dati), and purgative nut plant (nepala) should be pounded together, and after giving them the contact of the juice of the prickly plant (thor), pills should be made as large as one of gram. These pills will cure pain in the stomach.

2. Nine "tanks"[1] of oil if drunk remove pain in the stomach. One "pala"[1] of castor oil, two "palas" of . . . (words worn out) . . . should be drunk with ten "tanks"[1] of sugar to remove pain in the stomach.

3. Citrullus colocynthis (trush), black pepper, ten brinjals, seeds of castor oil plant, five good radishes, salt, carbonate of soda, bilvoben (sanchal), nitrate of potash, fifty leaves of thorn apple neutralised in the juice of cactus (thor) should be pounded together and put in a vessel. Then the process of Gujputmudra[2] should be done on them. The medicine should then be mixed with pepper, dill seeds, myrobalans, parsnip and bilvoben. After that the leaves of ark (ankdo) should be burnt and with the medicines named above should be rendered into ashes. These ashes will remove all kinds of stomach diseases: dropsy, colic, dyspepsia, and indigestion.

4. Half a pound of salt and two pounds of garlic should be burnt together by "putpak."[3] These two burnt should be mixed with bay breng (bidang), bilvoben

[1] *See* Appendix B—Weights.
[2] *See* Appendix A—Note II.
[3] *See* Appendix A—Note I.

(sanchal), salt and bambadoes aloes (kuver). These when taken with hot water remove shooting pains and flatulence.

5. A pound and a quarter of the five[1] kinds of salt (khar), half a pound of the flowers of ark (ankdo), one pound of bambadoes aloes (kuver) should be saturated with the juice of lemon and kept for 2 days underground. Powder should be made of these and eaten in the morning. By the use of this medicine all diseases of the stomach will be cured immediately.

6. Treacle, purging cassia (girmalo), pepper, turbeeth root (nasotar), chiretta, cloves, betel-nut, half a "tank"[2] of each and two "tanks" weight of myrobalans (abhaya) should be pounded together in the juice of the plant ocymum sanctum (tulshi), and ten pills should be made as large as a pod of pepper. These pills will cure all diseases of the stomach.

7. Bilvoben (sanchal), salt, myrobalans (abhaya), salt from sea water, nitrate of potash, bay breng (bidang), dry ginger, pepper, asafœtida, one "tank" weight of each; two pounds of carbonate of soda, eight "tanks" of parsnip should be powdered together and the powder taken in the morning for the removal of the pain in the stomach.

8. Having pounded the ten kinds of salt[3] (khar), tinospora cordifolia (galo) should be mixed with them. After eating this medicine treacle must be eaten and the pain in the stomach will vanish.

9. One pound of bambadoes aloes (kuver), thirty "tanks"[2] of salt-petre, bambadoes aloes purified in the juice of lemon and twenty nuxvomicas (jherkochlas) should be kept in whey for ten days. After ten days they should be placed on the fire for a short time, and the medicine thus prepared should be eaten in the morning. It cures all women's diseases following child-birth; cures dyspepsia, swelling and all diseases of the stomach.

[1] *See* Appendix A—Note III.
[2] *See* Appendix B—Weights.
[3] *See* Appendix A—Note IV.

XVII

PREPARATION OF THE SPECIFIC CALLED

SANKH-DRAV

(A solvent for dissolving shells)

Mineral salt, common salt, alum, and nitrate of potash should be pounded together with one "guna"[1] and half of salt-petre. They should be churned in a machine, then pure (sankh-drav) is obtained. It cures enlarged spleen, cancer and pain due to worms.

XVIII

THE OINTMENT CALLED

LOUSE—GUTI

1. Mollotus philippinensis (kapilo), sulphur, realgar (mansil) and a quantity of red lead (sindur) equal to all these should be properly mixed in oil. This ointment cures louse (guti).

2. A kind of gum which is applied to the wires of musical instruments to sharpen them (barjo) should be rubbed on a stone and then applied with the oil of the cashunut for the cure of louse.

XIX

IMPOTENCY IN MEN

1. Nutmeg, turmeric, dandelion (dudheli), colocynth (indravarna) and licorice (jethimadh) should be given with oil; this medicine removes impotency.

2. Seeds of colocynth (indravarna) should be pounded and made into a powder; that powder cures impotency.

[1] *See* Appendix B—Weights.

3. The skin of pomegranate should be finely powdered with resin and mixed with clarified butter (ghee) and then applied to the organ of generation to cure impotency.

4. Myrobalans, terminalia bellerica (beda), washed hogplums and gum should be applied with ficus glomerata (umber), ficus Bengalensia (vad) and butea frondosa (palash). After that red lead should be applied; this cures impotency.

XX

PURGATIVE MEDICINE

1. Mercury one "tank,"[1] sulphur one "tank," pepper one tank, borax (tankhankhar) one "tank," dry ginger one "tank," myrobalans (harade), one "tank," purgative nut plant (nepalo), seeds of the castor plant one "tank" should all be pounded together and the powder should be taken in hot water.

XXI

CURE OF

POISON OF A RABID DOG OR FOX

1. Lime, millet and salt should be bound together—as one binds dough—and soaked in the juice of the cactus plant and then made into cakes and they should be baked on the fire. They will act as a purgative, and the patient will be free from the effect of the poison.

2. Sugar candy, maize and myrobalans should be mixed with turbeeth root (nasotar) and should be taken in hot water. The patient will be purged and his bowels free.

3. Mysore gambostree (revanchi), natural ferri sulphate (geru) and cardemons should be taken with sugar candy; they will act as a purgative.

[1] *See* Appendix B—Weights.

XXII

WORMS

1. A combination of myrobalans (harade), terminalia bellerica (beda) and hogplums, oval-leaved rajabe (indrajava), mimosa catechu (kher), nimb tree fruit, sweet-flag root (vaj) should be prepared in the urine of a cow and drunk for the destruction of the worms in the stomach.

2. Curcuma zedooria (sadhi), solanum xanthocarpum (bharangi), simploces racemosa (lod), sweet-flag root (vaj), cassia occidentalis (kshundra), orris root (pushkarmul), pistachia integerrima (kakadsingi), pepper, chillies, myrobalans, salt, bilvoben (sanchal), cyrapus rotundas (moth), should be powdered together and made into large pills in honey; these pills will destroy the bag of worms in the stomach.

3. Pepper root, myrobalans, costus root, asafœtida, bilvoben, salt and turbeeth root (nasotar) will kill all worms in the stomach.

XXIII

PAIN IN THE EAR

1. Turbeeth root (nasotar), pepper, bay breng (vavading), (banulkham), the juice of all in equal proportion, dropped in the ear, remove ear-ache.

2. Juice of the horseradish tree, honey and oil should be heated on the fire and dropped into the ear.

3. The juice of all the four substances: clerodendron phlomoides (arno), jambu, Indian lilace tree (nimb tree) and costus root (kuth) should be obtained and mixed with oil and dropped into the ear. The pain will be removed.

4. Gall nut (majufal), pepper and alum should be powdered and blown into the ear.

5. Garlic should be fried in the oil of synapis alba (katu oil) and two or four drops of that oil should be poured into the ear.

6. Salt, dry ginger, sweet-flag root, dill seeds, asafœtida (ramath), cedar (devdar) and costus root (kuth) should be powdered and mixed in the urine of a she-goat. This medicine removes pain in the ear.

7. Salt melted in the urine of a goat should be poured in the ear.

8. Powder of the ashes of cowries should be soaked in the juice of a lemon. This also cures pain in the ear.

9. A leaf of the gigantic solvert (ankda) tree should be smeared with clarified butter (ghee) and salt and these should be baked in that leaf. The juice of that leaf should then be expressed and used as drops for the ear.

10. The juice of cephalondra Indica (tindori) and pepper remove the pain of the ear. Acacia catechu (khar), carbonate of soda (sachoro) melted in the juice of lemon should be dropped into the ear.

11. Horseradish tree (saradhu) and treacle should be crushed together and mixed with the juice of lemon. These drops remove the pain in the ear.

12. The seeds of the thorn apple, sulphur, Indian mazorian (girani), seeds of solanum xanthocarpum (kshundra) should be pounded together and mixed with the oil of sweet-flag root and sandal.

13. Salt, cyrapus rotundas (moth), cenabar (hingalo), dry ginger, bilvoben (sanchal), nitrate of potash, sweet-flag root, carbonate of soda and cedar should be pounded together and then they should be boiled with salt, horse-radish tree, ginger, garlic and cytrus medica (bijora) in oil. This oil is a very good medicine for ear-ache.

XXIV

PARTIAL HEADACHE

(ADHASHISHI—Literally half headache)

1. By inhaling the vapour of hot water in which salt, pepper and realgar (mansil) have been boiled, the headache will be cured.

2. Headache is cured by inhaling the vapour of the oil in which synapis alba (sarasav), carbonate of soda, sweet-flag root, urine of the cow, asafœtida and bay breng (vavading) have been boiled.

3. Partial headache is cured by inhaling the vapour of the water in which country soap nut (aritha) has been boiled; and it is also cured by inhaling the vapour of water in which are boiled treacle and dry ginger.

4. By anointing the nose with lime and dry ginger, white and black pepper pounded together, the headache is cured.

XXV

GUINEA WORMS—VALA

1. Salt, opium, soap, garlic, asafœtida and thorn apple should be crushed together and applied to the affected part of the body; and a piece of cloth tied over it. The disease will be cured.

2. Asafœtida, the horn of a deer (sabarsing), carbonate of soda, turmeric, soap, opium, all crushed and bandaged on the affected part of the body remove guinea worms.

3. Tender sprouts of the castor oil plant, prickly plant (dhuvas-dhamaso) and carbonate of soda should be crushed together and bound on the affected part of the body to cure guinea worms.

4. Having crushed the leaves of mustard pods (raysang) apply a paste of them on the affected part and over them a paste of the medicines already named. By doing so, the patient will feel coolness, his pain will vanish and the guinea worms will not remain in the body.

XXVI

SWELLING—SHOFF

1. Dry ginger, Indian lilace-tree leaves, cedar, turmeric myrobalans (abhaya), hellebore nigrum (katu), tinospora cordifolia (galo), and new trichosanthe dioica (patol) boiled together make a very good poultice for the swelling.

2. Cyrapus rotundas (moth), trichosanthe cucumerina (patol), the root of the brinjal tree, myrobalans terminalia bellerica (beda), and hogplums, cedar, turmeric, hellebore nigrum (katu), the inner bark of the Indian lilace tree all in equal proportion with two " tanks " of bdellium (guggal) should be boiled together to make a poultice for swelling or the wind which causes swelling.

3. Having well rubbed the body with the juice of macuna pruriens (makadi), a combination of myrobalans, terminalia bellerica and hogplums, cyrapus rotundas (moth), Persian lilace, plumbago zeylanica (chitrak), clerodendron phlomoids (arani), and the three-leaved chaste tree (nigod) should be boiled and given to the patient to be drunk. It removes melancholia mandukva.

4. The patient suffering from swelling (shoff) in the stomach should first take a purgative, afterwards drinking the urine of the cow for nine days. It cures the swelling in the stomach.

XXVII

STRICTURE OF THE URETHRA—MUTRAKRUCHHA

1. Five "tanks" of nitrate of potash should be divided into fourteen parts. Each part should be taken with whey daily. It will cure stricture of the urethra.

2. Treacle and turmeric should be taken in equal proportion with a gruel of corn (kanji). It will cure this disease.

3. Fruit pulp of purging cassia (gir), purging cassia (girmalo), padellium muracus (gokhru), myrobalans (abhaya), camel thorn (javas) should be boiled together and drunk with honey; it will cure this disease.

4. By eating sugar, grapes and cream of the curdled milk this disease will be cured.

5. It is also cured by eating the white substance of the bamboo (vans-lochan), sugar candy, padellium muracus (gokhru) with clarified butter (ghee).

6. It is also cured by drinking a tea made from cardemons saxifraga ligulata (bhed), honey, pepper, padellium muracus (gokhru) and "shilajit"[1] with treacle.

7. Pepper, myrobalans, hogplums, cyrapus rotundas (moth), licorice, "shilajit," sugar candy, padellium muracus (gokhru) all should be powdered and the powder eaten.

8. Excretions of mice should be put in the navel of the suffering person, and treacle and milk should be drunk.

For the benefit of students these verses have been simply composed. I request the wise to appreciate them.[2]

[1] NOTE.—"Shilajit" is a black astringent preparation well known in India. It is collected from stones by a method known to few. The translator learnt the process from the French Sadhu, the late Bawa Mast Ram Mahant of Jakko Temple, Simla.

[2] This naïve note has been kept in its place.

XXVIII

SWELLING AND ULCER OF THE MOUTH—MUKH-PAK

1. Take an equal proportion of cedar (devdar), turmeric, a combination of myrobalans, terminalia bellerica and hogplums, amsepida ball (kayfal), licorice, grapes, trichosanthe cucumerina (patol) and have them boiled in water and keep that water in the mouth.

XXIX

ECTHYMA—VISFUTAK

NOTE.—This disease is caused by intercourse with harlots and low women.

1. Mercuras sulphide (kajali) should be made from mercury, " sar," and sulphur (gandhak) mixed with twenty " tanks " of butter. This medicine cures ecthyma.

2. Two " tanks " of white sublimate (ras-kapur) and four " tanks " of sugar candy should be divided into fourteen parts; these 14 parts taken for seven days, twice daily, cure this disease.

3. White sublimate (ras-kapur) one " tank," cloves and pepper each 20 in number, should be pounded together and divided into seven parts. This medicine will cure ecthyma.

4. Cloves, plumbago zeylanica (chitrak), cenabar (hingalo) should be taken in equal proportion, and a third of their weight of realgar (mansil) should be mixed with them; they should be kept on the live coals formed from the wood of acacia catechu -(khadir) and their smoke should be taken on the body. The boils will disappear.

5. Smoke of oval-leaved rajabe (indrajava), opium (safain), cenabar (hingalo), plumbago zeylanica (chitrak),

purple goat's rue (sarpankho), and yellow orpiment (harital) will also cure ecthyma.

6. Solanum xanthocarpum (kshundra), realgar (mansil), cenabar, white clay (gopi-chandan), calcium sulphide (godanta), plumbago zeylanica (chitrak), aloes (elah) all should be powdered and divided into fourteen parts.

7. Smoke of red sulphide of mercury (hingalo), and shells of poppy (posat), each two "tanks," should be used for fumigating the body, carefully covering the eyes, for three days.

8. The smoke from live coals of the acacia catechu tree (khadir) also cures the boils of ecthyma.

9. Pepper root and clarified butter (ghee) and their weight of camphor (kapur) also cure ecthyma.

10. A pill made of argemone mexicana (chokh), the purgative nut plant (nepala), red sulphide of mercury (hingalo), each one "masa"[1] in weight taken in treacle for seven days cures ecthyma.

XXX

CARBUNCLE—PATHA

1. Adiantum lunulatum (hanspadi)—a vegetable—fried in ghee should be applied on the carbuncle for seven days. The patient will be all right.

2. Having rubbed bones of different kinds on a stone with water, the carbuncle should be anointed with the paste for seven nights; by doing so, no trace of the carbuncle will remain.

3. The dung of pigs should be burnt and a quarter of a pound of these ashes should be passed through a sieve of fine cloth. These ashes (quarter of a pound) should be pounded together with six "tanks" of lawsonia inermis (mendi) and mixed with oil. This medicine should be applied for twenty-one days. It cures even scrofula.

[1] *See* Appendix B—Weights.

4. Dead musk-rat (chachhunder) applied with oil cures this disease immediately.

5. Leaves of mustard (raysang) should be crushed and this lump should be tied on the carbuncle. The process should be repeated 21 times and then the disease will be cured.

6. Bones of a camel should be burnt and an ointment should be prepared of them in clarified butter (ghee). This ointment when applied to the carbuncle will cure the disease.

XXXI

WHITLOW—KHILLI

1. Lime, treacle, roots of kuskus grass (chhalak); all these should be crushed together and made into a lump. That lump should be tied on the whitlow; it will be cured.

2. The flowers of the gigantic solvert (ankda) tree and leaves of the tamarind tree should be boiled; and these hot flowers and leaves of tamarind with their vapour should be bound on the whitlow with clay. After this poultice, salt and butter should be smeared on the whitlow. The whitlow will be cured.

3. A poultice should be made of the flower of wheat and salt in the juice of the gigantic solvert (ankda) tree. It should be tied on the finger. The whitlow will subside.

XXXII

BURNS

If á person is burnt by fire, water, clarified butter (ghee), or oil, the following are the medicines :—

1. Juice of the banyan tree with sesamum oil should be anointed on the body.

2. Poppy seeds (khaskhas), resin (ral) and costus root (kath) should be powdered and passed through a fine cloth. Then they should be mixed with oil and the ointment thus prepared should be applied.

3. Seeds of the castor oil plant (arand) should be ground in the milk of an ewe. This ointment should be applied to the spots.

4. Milk from the female breasts should be first anointed and over this the powder of myrobalans should be sprinkled. By it the pain will be removed and the patient will feel happy.

5. The dung of a she-goat and the stones or kernels of green dates should be burnt together, and then mixed with oil; the juice of the cactus should be applied to the burnt spots.

XXXIII

NOSE-BLEEDING

1. Roots of cynodon dactylon (dhro-durva) and juice of the mango tree and milk and sugar should be drunk to stop nose-bleeding.

2. Terminalia chebula (harmaj), antimony (sarma), simploces racemosa (lod), the juice of the green bamboo, anglea roxburghiana (ghaunla) should be taken with honey; the blood will then stop flowing.

3. Terminalia chebula (harmaj), antimony (sarma), simploces racemosa (lod), a combination of myrobalans, terminalia bellerica and hogplums, juice of "katjan" should be kept in clarified butter (ghee) and then that medicine should be eaten.

4. Cumin seeds (jira), and the flowers of pomegranate should be crushed together with sugar candy. Pills made of these stop the blood coming into the mouth.

5. Fruit pulp of feronia elephantum (kuthvadi), sugar, hogplums, the juice of adhatoda vasica (vasa) resin (ral) all pounded together stop the blood coming into the mouth.

6. Poerhavia verticillatch (pat-khaparyo) and cardemons should be powdered and made into pills with clarified butter (ghee). Three of these pills stop the blood flowing.

XXXIV

PEENUS—OZÆNA

1. Peenus (ozæna) is cured by black pepper with treacle and curds. Peenus is also cured by inhaling the vapour of the water in which treacle and dry ginger are boiled together.

2. Peenus is cured by applying dry ginger and lime of shells (chhip) on the nose.

3. The nose should be washed with water in which the crushed powder of black pepper and luffa achinata (bindali) is thrown.

4. A mixture of the combination of myrobalans, terminalia bellerica (beda) and hogplums, honey and pepper should be taken and water should be drunk afterwards through the nose.

5. Salt and oil should be pounded together and boiled afterwards; this vapour should be inhaled through the nose; thus, the peenus is cured.

XXXV

LEUCORRHŒA

(Pradra disease of women)

1. Senna (sonamukhi), sprouts of the mango tree, sandal, roots of lotus, water in which rice is washed should be taken to cure leucorrhœa.

2. Sandal, the white substance found in the bamboo, cumin seeds, sugar, resin and water in which rice is washed cure this disease.

3. Pot herb (tandaljo) and casalpinia bonducella (kankachi) should be powdered with their roots; this powder when eaten stops leucorrhœa.

4. Sugar and mint (fuddi) each two "tanks" should be mixed with treacle and clarified butter (ghee) and pills should be made of them.

5. Coriander seeds (sokh), scirpus kysoor (kasel), Bengal maderroots (majith) should be pounded together in the juice of the dandelion (dudheli) and a lump of them should be put in the vagina; it cures the disease of leucorrhœa.

6. Corchorus antichorus (bahufali), the flowers of butea frondosa (khakhra) tree, hygrophila spinosa (akhro), with the skin of the pomegranate should be powdered and powdered sugar equal to the weight of this powder should be mixed with it. This powder should be drunk in cow's milk.

7. Flour of vetch and a kind of grain named "adab" with hornbeam-leaved cedar (balbeej), gum, clarified butter (ghee) and good rice eaten in the morning cures white leucorrhœa.

8. White leucorrhœa is also cured by eating lakh (lac), resin, terminalia bellerica (beda), and mesna ferrea (nagkeshar) all in equal proportion with sugar.

9. Leucorrhœa is cured by eating the powder of terminalia bellerica (beda), hygrophila spinosa (akhro), hogplums, greaslia tomentoza (dhavdi), cumin seeds (jeera), coriander seeds (sokh), sugar and the fruit pulp of feronia elephantum (kuthkivdi).

10. The excretion of the wild dove (kapot) with rice-water stops the flowing of the blood.

11. The excretion of mice and hogplums should be eaten with sugar.

XXXVI

REMOVAL OF HAIR

1. Having drawn out the hair of the vagina, the seeds of trichosanthus cucumerina (patola-beej), boiled in oil should be anointed in the vagina. The hair will not again grow there.

XXXVII

DISEASES OF WOMEN AFTER CHILDBIRTH

1. Two "pals"[1] of winter cherries (asandh), four pounds of rice, one "pal" of dry ginger, and white and black pepper, should be fried and clarified butter (ghee) and sugar should be mixed with them after taking them down from the fire.

By eating this medicine diseases of women after childbirth (suva-rog) are cured.

2. Two "pals"[1] of white sesamum with dry ginger, cumin seeds and parsnip all together eight "tanks" in weight should be pounded, and the patient should begin by taking two "tanks" and increase them up to twelve "tanks"; the "suva-rog" will be cured.

3. Sugar, licorice and the seeds of lotus (kand-kaj) also cure "suva-rog"

XXXVIII

PAIN IN THE VAGINA

1. Three "tanks" of the roots of alhagi moururum (javaso) should be drunk in cold water.

[1] *See* Appendix B—Weights.

2. Yellow leaves of the cotton tree should be pounded and formed into a pill which should be put in the vagina; afterwards the juice of hogplums, together with the leaves of the pot-herb (cholai) should be applied. The pain will vanish.

3. The fruits of the thorn apple (dhatura), dry ginger (nagar), costus root (kuth) should be ground and made into a syrup or kanji. When it is hot, it should be anointed on the navel; the pain will vanish.

XXXIX

WARTS (MASA) IN THE VAGINA

If there are warts in the vagina, heat should be applied to the vagina with an earthen pot.

1. Camphor, gallnut, quercus infectorius (mangfal), alum (turi), paleteri root (marhatti) should be crushed and anointed on the warts. These should be applied with the hands for seven days, during which time the disease will be cured.

XL

MALODOROUS VAGINA

1. Having boiled the leaves of the Indian lilace tree (nimb), these leaves with camphor should be applied to the vagina after washing. The bad odour will vanish.

2. Costus root (uplet), camphor, aloe-wood (agar), kuskus grass (usir), flour of gram and oil should be rubbed on the body. The odours of the body will vanish.

XLI

BURNING SENSATION IN THE VAGINA

1. Powder of the skin of pomegranate, quarter of a pound of alum equal to two rupees in weight, licorice (jethimadh) equal to half a rupee in weight; these three should be pounded, passed through a sieve and drunk with quarter of a pound of water. By drinking it the burning sensation in the vagina will subside.

2. Salt, cumin seeds (jeera), licorice (jethimadh), aniseeds (variyali), and skin of pomegranate should all be passed through a sieve and mixed with an equal proportion of sugar. The pills made from them will cure burning sensation in the vagina.

XLII

CONTRACTION OF THE VAGINA

1. A combination of myrobalans, terminalia bellerica (beda) and hogplums, gallnut, alum, tamarix gallica (padvas), scirpus kysoor (kasel) all should be pounded together and the pill made of them should be kept in the vagina.

2. Salt, skin of pomegranate both in equal proportion, should be crushed together; their pill should be kept in the vagina and there should be no sexual intercourse.

3. Myrobalans (abhaya), gallnut, alum, terminalia chebula (harmaj), the gum of the red silk cotton tree (mochrasa), tamarix gallica (padvas), tamarind, green vitriol (hirakashi) and flowers of jasmine (jhaḥi) all should be crushed and a pill of these kept in the vagina.

4. The powder of alum and gallnut is efficacious for the vagina.

5. Fœungreek grass (methi), alum, simploces racemosa (lodra), and tamarix gallica (padvas) should be powdered; this powder kept in the vagina destroys water.

6. Alum, terminalia chebula (harmaj), gallnut, greaslia tomentoza (dhave) all should be powdered; this powder should be kept in the vagina for contraction.

XLIII

UT PRIUS EMITTAT MULIER

1. Membro virili in coitu camphore aloque enuncto prius ejaculat mulier.

2. Membro virili nuce mangonio Indicæ triturato enuncto statim ejaculat mulier.

3. Pudendo prius floribus tamaricis plumbo rubro camphore melique contritis enuncto statim orgasmum perdit mulier.

XLIV

UT ERIGAT MEMBRUM VIRILE

1. Cannibus sativa (bhang), the root of gigantic solvert (ankdo) tree and sweet-scented oleander (karana) and the seeds of the thorn apple (dhatura) should all be pounded together, and dried in the shade. Having crushed them in the urine of a male, quibus enunctum, membrum sese quam maxime extendit roburat erigit.

XLV

FOR MAKING A WOMAN'S BREASTS HARD

1. The breasts should be smeared with an ointment made of the root of the sweet-scented oleander (karana-kaner), costus root (kuth), peppera longa (gajkarana), sweet-flag root (vaj) and winter cherries (asandh) ground together for making them hard.

XLVI

AMAN-ANI-RECTI

1. Aman (recti) is replaced in its natural position by giving to it for five days the smoke of red woollen cloth and realgar (mansil) pounded with pandanus foscicularis (ketaki).

2. Recti (aman) is replaced by pressing it with a piece of copper plate smeared with butter and the crushed flowers of greaslia tomentoza (dhavdi).

XLVII

PILES

1. Carbonate of soda, the lime used in betel leaves, and salt, all in equal proportion should be ground in the juice of lemon. By applying this medicine to the piles, the disease will be removed.

2. The piles will be removed by smearing them with an ointment made of saltish earth (khara) ground down in water.

3. Green vitriol (hirakashi), and alum, ground down in water and applied destroys piles.

4. Carbonate of soda, lime, yellow orpiment (hartal) and borax (tankankhar) should be powdered together, and after passing them through a sieve, they should be boiled. By applying this medicine, piles are removed.

XLVIII

WHITE LEPROSY

1. Three "tanks"[1] of bilvoben (sanchal), twenty "tanks" of the ashes of shells (chhip), one "tank" of

[1] *See* Appendix B—Weights.

nitrate of potash, three "tanks" of turmeric should be passed through a fine cloth and then ground together in shilarasa-shilajit.[1]

This medicine should be applied to the body after the oil of jasmine (chambeli) is applied. It will remove the white spots from the skin.

2. After applying the powder of the Indian lilace (nimb) tree, the skin should be washed with the water of the babul tree; white spots will disappear and the skin will be in good condition.

3. Gunja (chanothi), lemon, costus root (kuth), sweet-flag root (vaj), plumbago zeylanica (chitrak) all should be pounded together and made into an ointment in whey. By applying this ointment white spots will disappear.

4. Purgative nut plant (ajepal) and cow dung should be boiled together and then applied to the skin. Over this powdered myrobalans, terminalia bellerica (beda) and hogplums should be sprinkled; the white spots will disappear.

5. Thorn apple (dhaturo), sweet-scented oleander (kanera-kaner), cactus (thor), sprouts of jasmine (jai), pongunia globra (karanj), resin (saram-ras), plumbago zeylanica (chitrak) should all be boiled in oil and rubbed on the body.

6. Indian jalup (nishot), conscura decussata (chandgan), hogplums and myrobalans should be powdered and their pills should be made in treacle. They should be taken for twenty-one days. They cure even the leprosy in which pus comes out of the body and where limbs decay.

7. Brinjal (bengan), troiling eclipta (bhangaro) one pound, calcium sulphide (godant), iron (loha) and pepper should be passed through the process of "putpak"[2] and then applied.

8. Four pounds of lime should be given the "bhavna"[3]

[1] See Note Page 33.
[2] *See* Appendix A—Note III.
[3] *See* Appendix A—Note II.

of the juice of leea robessta (kakjungha) and the juice of bambadoes aloes (kuver) and should then be placed in an earthen pot. The pot should be covered with a lid or an earthen cover, and the mouth of the earthen pot with that cover should be made air-tight with quick lime (chunam). The pot should be placed underground, and covered with sand up to its mouth. It should be heated by fire for nine hours and then heated in the middle for six hours. After thus giving it heat for 21 hours, the vessel should be taken out. The fire must be without smoke, and only when smokeless should the medicine be placed on the fire. This medicine should be given equal in weight to half a " gunja " (chanothi)[1] with cold water.

XLIX

SYPHILIS, BOILS AND ULCERS

(Which are not healed easily)

1. Bell-tree fruit (beela), betel-nuts, poparlind fig tree (pipalo), cactus (thuhar), achyrontches aspera (aghadi), bones of a goat, skull of a man, all these seven things should be burnt into ashes. Lime, bdellium (guggal), blue vitriol, catechu, bulb of lotus (kaselo), mixture of mercury and sulphur (kajali) should be ground together with the ashes mentioned before. This medicine should be pounded in clarified butter (ghee) in a copper vessel and then applied to the diseased parts; by this even the syphilis which is not healed, with all boils and ulcers, boils which are filled with pus that burst and are again filled with pus (bharnigal) are cured.

2. Ulcers on the breasts of women, ulcers on the legs, scrofula (kanthmal), fistula (nasur), ulcers on the head, and scurvy (kharjva) are also cured by this medicine.

[1] *See* Appendix B—Weights.

3. Blue vitriol, resin, catechu and turmeric should be ground together in oil and water. This medicine cures all kinds of boils, pimples, ulcers and poisoning from marking nuts (bhilama).

4. Mollotus philippinensis (kapilo), catechu of ten " tanks " weight, lime eight " tanks," red lead one " tank," pepper and blue vitriol eight " tanks " should be pounded together and smeared with caledupa arborea (karanj) oil. This medicine will cure ulcers which are not easily healed.

5. Resin, costus root (kuth), honey-comb wax (kashikath), clarified butter (ghee) and wax with a quarter of a pound of hogplums should all be burnt to ashes. These ashes with cassia tora (punvad), fat of pig (charmi-barah), chimney smoke deposits (dhuso), one " tank " of pepper and one " tank " of blue vitriol should be finely crushed in the clarified butter (ghee) of the cow and then applied to syphilis or ulcers ; they will be cured immediately.

6. Mollotus philippinensis (kapilo), litharge (or) massicot (murdarsingdi), gallnut, red lead, bdellium (guggal), natural ferri sulphate (geru), resin one " tank " should be powdered. Then four " tanks " of wax should be heated with clarified butter (ghee). The powder of these medicines should be thrown into this heated wax and clarified butter (ghee) and the medicine thus prepared applied to the unhealed spots which will be cured.

7. Cordia latifolia (gundi), with green leaves, should be reduced to ashes which should weigh five " tanks." These ashes with half a " tank " each of chillies, blue vitriol, cashunut and catechu should be powdered in the oil of synapis alba (sarasav) on a plate. This medicine should be applied to the unhealed spots.

8. Mollotus philippinensis (kapilo), gum, litharge (or) massicot, resin, red lead each of two " tanks " weight, camphor quarter of a " tank," blue vitriol and alum one

"tank" should all be powdered and mixed with the wax of a honey-comb; this medicine should be applied to the unhealed spots. It cures all boils and pimples.

9. Blue vitriol, red lead, resin, each of the weight of two "tanks," catechu, one "tank," and litharge (or) massicot (bodar), three "tanks" should be powdered and mixed with heated clarified butter and wax. This medicine should be applied to the boils of syphilis, or other boils, and they will be cured.

COUGH OF CONSUMPTION

1. Three "tanks" of dry ginger and one "tank" of opium should be powdered together and made into pills as large as pepper. This medicine removes this cough.

2. The fruit of the thorn apple (dhatura) should be split crossways and filled with salt. Having smeared it with dung, it should be baked in the fire. When it is cool, it should be eaten with sugar in the morning in the measure of two "turas"[1] only. The coughing will be cured.

3. Pepper, calcium sulphide (godanti), realgar (mansil), blue vitriol, bdellium (guggal) should be pounded in the juice of the gigantic solvert (ark) and pills as large as a gram should be made of that powder. This pill should be placed on the fire and the smoke of that pill should be swallowed by means of a tube placed in the mouth in the manner of a person smoking. The cough will be cured.

4. Casalpinia bonducella (kuber), pepper, salt, good kind of dry ginger equal in all to quarter of a pound should be powdered. This powder and 40 leaves of the gigantic solvert (ankdo) tree should be placed in an earthen pot. Then ten "pals"[1] of solanum xanthocarpum (kshundra)

[1] *See* Appendix B—Weights.

should be taken and one brinjal with the solanum xanthocarpum (kshundra) should be placed in that earthen pot. The pot should then be closed and heated. Two "tanks" of the medicine thus prepared should be given for curing cough and asthma.

5. An equal proportion of pistachia integerrima (singi), dry ginger, pepper, orris root (pushkarmul), zelory (kachoor), cyrapus rotundas (moth), clerodendron serratum (bharangi), and black pepper should be powdered, and by eating that powder cough is cured.

6. Adhatoda vasica (vasa), dry ginger, pepper, all the three, in equal proportion, should be powdered together and pills should be made in honey for the cough.

7. Five fruits of colocynth (indravarna), five brinjals, five bambadoes aloes (kunver), fifty fruits of solanum xanthocarpum (kshundra), ten fruits of thorn apple (kanak), ten leaves of gigantic solvert (ark), one pound and a half of casalpinia bonducella (kuber), five pounds and a quarter of salt; all these should be powdered and spread in an earthen pot. Then the process of "gajputmudra"[1] should be applied to that pot. One "tank" of the medicine thus prepared taken in the morning with sesamum cures swelling, asthma, consumption, pain in the stomach, anæmia and indigestion.

LI

CONSUMPTION

1. Borax (tankhan) and alum which is swollen or heated and eaten with betel leaf, cures the cough of consumption, and the weight of the patient is increased.

2. Consumption is cured by eating in betel leaf the juice of post-bau, and arsenic equal to half a grain of rice.

[1] *See* Appendix A—Note I.

LII

BAD SMELL IN THE MOUTH

1. After brushing the teeth with powdered tobacco keep cumin seeds (jeera) in the mouth ; the bad smell of the mouth will be removed.

2. Nutmeg (jatifal), cardemons, and cinnamon should be powdered and made into a pill. By keeping that pill in the mouth, the bad smell will vanish.

3. Flour of gram, cloves, cardemons, mesna ferrea (nagkeshar) and camphor should be rubbed on the body with water to remove the bad smell of the body.

LIII

TOOTHACHE

1. The skin of winter cherries (asandh) and their roots and fœun-greek grass (methi) should be kept in the cheeks to remove toothache.

2. A pill made of borax (tankhan) and pepper should be kept in the hollow of the aching tooth.

3. Blue vitriol and alum swollen on fire should be kept in the mouth to remove toothache.

4. Pepper and seeds of solanum xanthocarpum (kshudra) should be pounded together and their pills should be made in the juice of cactus (thuhar). This pill removes toothache.

5. A kind of gum (kamato), country soapnut (aritha) should be powdered and made into pills. This pill should be kept in the hollow of the aching tooth. It gives instantaneous relief.

6. Gallnut (maju), catechu, pepper, salt, simploces racemosa (lod) should be powdered and put into the

aching tooth and gallnut (maju) and parsnip (ajmo) should be rubbed on it.

7. Hellebore nigrum (kadu), costus root (kuth), adhatoda vasica (vasa), catechu, simploces racemosa (lod), Bengal maderroots (majith) should be powdered in the clarified butter (ghee) and put into the aching tooth to remove pain.

LIV

FOR MAKING THE COMPLEXION FAIR

1. Costus root (uplot), synapis alba (sarasav), mustard each one "tank" in weight and cumin seeds (jeerak) twice as much as these in all should be boiled in milk and applied to the face for making the complexion fair.

2. A soup (kanji) should be prepared of turmeric and synapis alba (sarasav) and applied to the face, and pills made of saffron should be eaten for making the complexion fair.

3. Turmeric and almonds should be ground down with milk and applied to the face.

4. By applying the soup (kanji) of turmeric and cumin seeds (jeerak) a dark complexion is made fair.

LV

PIMPLES ON THE FACE

1. Dry ginger, salt, simploces racemosa (lodra), sweet-flag root (vaj) all in equal proportion should be pounded together in water and applied to the pimples for removing them.

2. Dry ginger . . . words worn out . . . should be rubbed on a stone in water and applied to the pimples to remove them. No trace of them will be left on the face.

LVI

FISTULA OF THE NOSE—NASUR

1. Cloves, pepper, byrangtonia acuteangula (samudrafal) should be rubbed on a stone with water and applied to the fistula. It will be cured.

2. Red ochre (geru), turmeric (nisha), red sandalwood (ratanjali), the powder of an old brick, seeds of rayan fruit . . . words worn out . . . should be ground with milk and applied to fistula.

3. Sprouts of cappasis aphylla (kerada) and juice of berberis aristata (raswanti) should be ground together and applied to the fistula.

4. The horn of a buffalo should be burnt and its ashes, mixed with butter, should be applied to the fistula. By this medicine the hole will soon close up.

5. A human skull should be powdered with cow dung and mixed with clarified butter (ghee). It should then be applied to the fistula ; the hole will be closed.

LVII

EXCESSIVE MICTURITION

1. Nine " tanks " each of dry ginger, white and black pepper and burnt gram should be made into pills in treacle. These pills should be eaten for three days for excessive micturition.

2. Pepper, thorn apple (kana), mixed with three times more in weight than the pepper of clarified butter (ghee) and paleteri root (akalkaro) should be made into pills. A pill should be taken in the evening after making water. It stops nocturnal emissions.

LVIII

GONORRHŒA

Twenty kinds of Gonorrhœa are caused by excess of fat and flesh, cough, heat (ushna), bile, lymph (ras), bone marrow and excessive lasciviousness.

Names of Gonorrhœa

(1) Ikshu	(8) Aruldiyo
(2) Baluk	(9) Kshar
(3) Udak Ras	(10) Majith
(4) Lavona	(11) Haladio
(5) Shartara	(12) Neelmasi
(6) Badhya-prasta	(13) Rakta
(7) Takra	

All these are caused by bile (pitta) and are difficult to cure.

(14) Ghrita	(16) Hasti
(15) Madhu	(17) Vasu

These are caused by wind (vayu) and are incurable.

LIX

MEDICINES

1. By drinking five "tanks" of the juice of pomegranate and sugar equal to one pice in weight gonorrhœa (red premeha), in which there is burning sensation, is cured.

2. Fourteen "tanks" of the juice of lemon should be mixed with one pound of water. In it natural ferri sulphate (shankhgeru) should be thrown, and the medicine thus prepared should be given to cure gonorrhœa.

3. Three "tanks" of treacle, mixed with the whey from cow's milk, cure gonorrhœa.

4. The leaves of tamarind (ambli) remove the burning sensation and give happiness to the body. Country babul tree brush (datan) . . . words worn out . . .

5. Gonorrhœa is cured by drinking the flowers of the babul tree crushed with sugar candy.

6. Adiantum lunulatum (handspadi), cumin seeds (jeera), asparagopsis racemosus (shatvari), feronia elephantum (koth), parsnip (ajmo), iron (loh), cardemons (alayachi), calcium sulphate (pakhan), and boerhavia diffusa (punarnava) also cure gonorrhœa.

7. Mesna ferrea (nagkeshar), asparagus ascendens (musali), starch of tinaspora cordifolia (amarsatva), winter cherries (asandh), and sugar should be powdered and made into pills with honey. These pills cure red gonorrhœa.

8. Bengal maderroots (majith), gallnut (maju), padellium muracus (gokhru), a combination of myrobalans, terminalia bellerica (beda) and hogplums each five "tanks" with honey cure red gonorrhœa (rakta prameha).

9. Ten tanks of turmeric, hogplums twice as much in weight, i.e., twenty "tanks," taken with five "tanks" of lemon and sugar cure "haladi" gonorrhœa (haladi prameha).

10. Hygrophila spinosa (akhro), adhatoda vasica (vasa), padellium muracus (gokhru), myrobalans, terminalia bellerica (beda) and hogplums, pudding pipe tree or purging cassia (girmalo), acacia catechu (kher), turmeric (nisha) and cedar (devdar) cure gonorrhœa (madhu prameha).

11. One "tank" of licorice (jethimadh) and seven "tanks" of sugar should be mixed with ghee and kept in ghee for twenty days. By eating this medicine daily as much as can be taken by a lick, gonorrhœa is cured.

12. Padellium muracus (gokhru), sugar, hogplums

(ambala), tinaspora cordifolia (amarsatva) should be eaten in honey to cure gonorrhœa.

13. Antimony (surma) and sugar should be pounded together and eaten to remove burning sensation when micturating (unva) and this medicine should be placed in the orifice of micturition.

14. Licorice (jethimadh), ox-gall (rochna), myrobalans, terminalia bellerica (beda) and hogplums and tobacco should be pounded together with sugar. This powder removes the pain of gonorrhœa.

END OF PART I

PART II

THE PROPER PLACES FOR BRANDING FOR THE CURE OF CERTAIN DISEASES[1]

1. Five inches (ten fingers) from the nose, there is the tenth opening (door); twenty fingers (angulas) in measurement from it there is the principal door (mul-dwar); fourteen fingers (angulas) from the principal door (mul-dwar) there is the waist; there are ten spots each ten fingers (angulas) distance from the nose.

2. By branding with a red-hot iron the spots half-an-inch to the right and the left of the heart, cough, hard-breathing and asthma will be cured.

3. "Cheena" is three-and-a-half inches from the heart and one inch to its right is the liver.

4. Five inches from the left there is the place of the enlarged spleen and half-an-inch from it is the spleen itself; that place is the place for the disease of "dhanuspyava" (tetanus).

The place should be kept warm; this disease is caused by impurity in the blood.

5. When the patient screams with pain and the body becomes cold, the symptoms indicate tetanus (dhanu-va).

[1] The translator herself saw this branding done by an expert with a red-hot clove, held in a pair of pincers when a case of wasting disease in a child, given up by the doctors, was cured. This art should be re-investigated.

Warmth should be applied to the middle of the spine (" bhur ").

Two inches away from that place, and three-fourths of an inch removed from the waist, the place should have heat applied or be branded.

6. For blood flowing from the nose and the mouth, or if the spleen is out of its place, a brand in the shape of a cross should be given at a spot one inch from the navel.

7. For delirium a brand should be given on the palate (talu), two brands on the temple and two should be given to the roots of the thumbs.

8. For headache and for toothache, a brand should be given to the roots of the thumbs and to the temples.

9. The toes of the feet should be branded (or heated) for sore eyes or sprue (galasi).

10. A round brand should be given on the hand in jaundice and on the " chima " for anæmia.

11. It should be given at a spot quarter of an inch removed from the lip for slow fever.

12. For enlarged spleen one brand should be marked on a place half-an-inch from the navel.

13. For enlargement of the testicles a brand on the palate.

14. In anæmia and sprue it should be given to the roots of the spine.

15. For insanity one on the belly, one cross-wise on " moor " (spine), one on the heart and two on the temples.

16. For the disease : retention of urine (mutrakrachha), one on the spot three-and-a-half inches below the navel; and for scrofula a brand should be given to a spot one inch above the navel.

17. For the pain of heart-failing a brand should be given at a spot two inches distance from the organ of generation (lingum).

II

BLOOD POISONING

(From the mauling of a Tiger.)

1. Lime, asafœtida, juice of the Indian lilace (nimb) tree, should be applied to the wound caused by the tiger, and the leaves of the nimb tree should be tied on it; the poison from the saliva of the tiger's mouth will be removed.

2. Asafœtida, pepper, cyrapus rotundas (moth), lime, Indian lilace (nimb) tree juice, bay breng (bidang), turmeric, asculint flacursia (babachi) all pounded together remove the poison of the tiger.

3. The juice of the nimb tree, asafœtida, lime, and pepper should be ground in the juice of cactus and the "bhavana"[1] of the juice of the gigantic solvert (ankdo) should be given to it. The pills made of these remove the poison of the tiger.

4. This pill of "Prabhavati" (medicine No. 3 above) should be rubbed in water and applied to the wound and the leaves of the nimb tree tied over it. The poison from the tooth of a tiger will be neutralised.

III

POISON OF A SERPENT

1. Winter cherries (asandh), the juice of castor plant, the juice of the pot-herb (cholai) should be drunk for the poison of a serpent. The poison is at once neutralised.

2. Half a "tank" of borax (tankhan) swollen on the fire should be given to a man, and on it he should be made to drink treacle and clarified butter (ghee). The poison of the snake will vanish.

[1] *See* Appendix A—Note III.

3. What can a serpent do to that man who takes borax only, equal to a seed of pepper, and drinks treacle and clarified butter (ghee) afterwards?

IV

POISON OF A MAD DOG OR JACKAL

1. The juice of the cactus should be given twice for the poison of a mad dog or a mad jackal.

WOUNDS

1. All kinds of wounds can be healed by anointing them with the roots of the babul tree pasted on a stone with water.

2. Simploces racemosa (lod), a combination of myrobalans, terminalia bellerica (beda) and hogplums, and thalictrum foliosum (tayman) should be pounded together and mixed with ghee. This medicine should be applied to the wound, and the leaves of the nimb tree should be boiled and tied on the wound. The wound is healed.

3. Mild Himalaya cherries (padmak), gymnosparia montana (vikaj), turmeric, hemidesmus Indicus (sariva), sandalwood (sukhad), simploces racemosa (lod), all in equal proportion, and each equal to one "pal"[1] should be boiled together in oil. The wound is healed when it is washed with this medicine, and also when the medicine is applied as a lotion.

4. Indian lilace (nimb), trichosanthe cucumerina (patol), costus root (uplot), berberis aristata (daru-haldar), the

[1] *See* Appendix B—Weights.

seeds of pongunia globra (karanja), wax, blue vitriol, Bengal meder roots (majith), myrobalans and clarified butter (ghee) equal to one "pal" should be boiled together. A decoction (quath) of them should be made; the wound being washed with this is at once healed, even if the wound is serious and there is hemorrhage.

5. Gum (gund), realgar (mansil), bdellium (guggal), blue vitriol, red lead (sindhur), asculint flacursia (babachi), and wax should be boiled and heated in clarified butter (ghee). The wound is healed by the application of this medicine.

VI

LOSS OF VITAL FLUIDS—DHATU

1. Piper cubeb (shitalchini), paleteri root (akalkaro), padellium muracus (gokhru), asparagus ascendens (musali), seeds of wild saffron (kasumbi), staff tree (kangni-malkangni), nutmeg (jatifal); all these are tonic medicines and prevent the loss of the vital fluids.

2. Mesna ferrea (nagkeshar), cardemons, spikenard valeriana (tagar), cinnamon (taj), saffron (kesar), cloves, cinnamon tomal (tamal-patra), the outer shell of nutmeg (javantri), mica-talc (abhrak), ashes of tin (bang-bhasma), orchis latifolia (salam), hygrophila spinosa (akhro), asparagus ascendens (musali), all in equal proportion, should be powdered and made into pills. The pills should be taken with honey, and milk should be drunk on them. This is an aphrodisiac.

3. Pepper root (granthik), dates, cyrapus rotundas (nagar-moth), sugar, honey and clarified butter (ghee) should be eaten in the morning and evening as a tonic or aphrodisiac.

4. One pound of the gum of acacia catechu (kher) and a preparation of wheat flour (nishasto) should be taken and the following medicines mixed with it :—

(1) Gygrophila spinosa (akhro),
(2) Padellium muracus (gokhru),
(3) Asparagus ascendens (musali),
(4) Seeds of macuna pruriens (kavuch),
(5) Orchis latifolia (salam),
(6) Cinnamon (taj),
(7) Buchanania latifolia (charoli),
(8) Nutmeg (jatifal),
(9) Outer shell of nutmeg (javantri),
(10) Cinnamon tomal (tamalpatra),
(11) Cloves (laving),
(12) Henbane (khurasan),
(13) Cannabis sativa (bhang),
(14) Black ocymum sanctum (black tulshi),
(15) The seeds of the Indian mello,
(16) Blepharis boerchaviafolia (utgan),
(17) Asparagus ascendens (musali),
(18) Cardemons (alachi),
(19) Palcteri root (akalkaro),
(20) China root (chopchini),
(21) Pepper: six "tanks" of each with poppy seeds (khaskhas) dates, dry ginger, almonds; all these should be powdered and the powder mixed with clarified butter (ghee) and treacle, and sweet balls should be made of them. If a person eats these sweet balls on rising his body will be very strong and healthy and have virility.

5. A pill made of snuff pounded in the juice of dry ginger if taken in the morning is a tonic and an aphrodisiac.

6. Half-a-pound of odourless asculint flacursia (bavachi) should be cut into pieces and five " tanks " of it should be boiled in a pound of milk and drunk daily.

7. Three " tanks " of poppy seeds and padellium muracus (gokhru) and sesamum equal to three " pice " in weight should be boiled in one pound of milk and gruel made. This gruel should be eaten in the evening to be strong and full of the virility of manhood.

8. Sugar, orchis latifolia (salam), and the gum of red silk cotton tree should be eaten boiled as a milk gruel for seven days to regain lost virility.

9. Padellium muracus (gokhru), macuna pruriens (kaucha), asparagus racemosus (satvari), cida spinosa (nagbal), cida cordifolia (balbeej), hygrophila spinosa (akhro), orchis latifolia (salam) taken with milk stops the loss of vital fluids.

10. Padellium muracus (gokhru), three-leaved chaste tree (nigadu), asparagus ascendens (musali), asparagus racemosus (satavari), winter cherries (aswagandh), macuna pruriens (kaucha), nutmeg (jayfal), cloves, cinnamon, cinnamon tomal (tamal), the skin of cida carpinifolia (gangeru) should all be taken in equal proportion and should be made into pills. This pill should be given with honey to restore potency.

11. White gourd (dudhi), corchorus antichorus (bahufali), should be crushed with water and drunk in the morning. And after that leaves of the " gundi " tree should be crushed and drunk in the same manner.

12. If a person boils seven " tanks " of onions in one pound and a half of milk and makes out of this a sort of curry and eats it standing for twenty-one days in the morning, he becomes strong, powerful and full of potency even if he is quite impotent.

VII

MEDICINE FOR RETENTIVE POWER

1. Sweet-scented oleander (kaner), jasminum grandiflorum (chambeli), gigantic solvert (ankdo), echinops echinatus (utkanto) the roots of each of these five things should be powdered, the combined powder weighing in all one " tank " only in weight. This powder should be thrown into one pound of milk which should be boiled until the whole turns into a pulp. A pill made from this pulp should be eaten with a quarter of a pound of sugar for retentive power.

2. Camphor, opium, nutmeg each weighing half a " tank," henbane (khorasan), bambadoes aloes (kunver) each weighing one " pice " should be powdered, and pills as large as a grain of gram should be made in oil. These pills should be given for retentive power.

3. Opium, sugar, nutmeg (jatifal), cenabar (hingalo), gum of odina nodier (bol), camphor, outer shell of nutmeg (javantri) should be powdered and pills made of them. This pill should be taken in a piece of lemon which should be sucked. This pill is very good for retention (sthambhan) and makes a man virile.

4. The root and skin of the sweet-scented oleander (kaner) and its flowers, pandanus foscicularis (ketaki) and hogplums two " tanks " each, paleteri root (akalkaro), each one " tank," should be powdered and pills made of them in the juice of gigantic solvert (ark). The ointment of this pill with saliva, quo enunctum foliis legatum, passionem per tres horas retinet membrum.

5. Nutmeg (jayfal), the outer shell of nutmeg (javantri), camphor, henbane (khorasan), casalpinia bonducella (kuber), saffron, sugar, opium, blepharis boerchaviafolia (utgan) should be taken in equal proportion and be pow-

dered. Pills should be made of this powder as large as a grain of gram. They are used for retentive power.

6. Opium and saffron should be taken in equal proportion and pills should be made of them. These pills placed in the orifice of the organ of generation give retentive power.

7. Camphor, saffron (kesar), nutmeg, henbale (khorasan), bambadoes aloes (kunver), paleteri root (akalkaro), thorn apple (dhaturo), parsnip (ajmo), cloves, blepharis boerchaviafolia (utgan), the root of white and red sweet-scented oleander padellium muracus (gokhru), myrobalans (abhaya), gallnut (manju) should be taken in equal proportion, powdered and made into pills. This pill eaten with milk and opium, vel in membri orificio insertum, holds Cupid, i.e., gives retention of vital fluids (sthambhan).

END OF PART II

PART III

CHARACTERISTICS OF A BARREN WOMAN

There are seven kinds of barren women and their barrenness is from seven different causes.

The first cause: The mouth of the womb (lotus) is upturned and cannot hold the fecundating seed.

The second cause: The mouth of the womb is sealed and the woman though intensely passionate cannot become pregnant. The remedy for this is as follows: A pill made of aloes with oil should be kept in the vagina.

The third cause: The mouth of the womb (lotus) is closed with warts. The remedy for this is cumin seeds, rice and aloes.

The fourth cause: Worms are produced in the womb. The remedy for this is a lump of pepper and opium placed in the mouth of the womb.

The fifth cause is due to too much heat in the womb so that the vital fluid of the male is burnt and the woman often gets prolonged monthly course. To cure this disease, barringtonia acuteangula (foam), pepper and camphor should be taken.

The sixth cause: The menstrual blood dries, and the blood will be cold; there will also be pain in the waist. The remedy is to smear pepper and aloes over the mouth of the womb.

The seventh cause is due to the work of some evil spirits who prevent the woman bearing a child. If a bud of sweet-scented oleander (kaner) is kept in the organ of the woman for fifteen hours (five yamas) and turns black that woman will never be able to bear a child.

If the vital fluid of the male placed in water sinks, it should be considered potent, i.e., able to produce a child; but if it floats on the water, it cannot produce offspring.

II

MEDICINE FOR THE BARRENNESS OF A WOMAN

1. Having judged from the appearance (limbs) of a woman, her characteristics, Yantra, Mantra and medicines should be carefully tried. First of all the woman should be given a purgative of turbeeth root (nisot) or purgative nut plant (nepala), one " tank " of each in sugar and milk for three days. This process should start in the days of the monthly course, and after this medicine rice and milk should be eaten. After taking this purgative, the remedies and medicines should be tried.

2. Mesna ferrea (nagkeshar), costus root (kuth), cumin seeds (jeera), cardemons, cinnamomum tomal (tamal-patra) should be powdered for four days. Fumigatory (pit-papado), ox-gall (gorochana), mesna ferrea (nag-keshar) and cloves should be taken with sugar candy for three days and milk should be drunk on them.

3. Mesna ferrea (nagkeshar) and excretions of wild pigeons, sugar candy and one seed of thespasia populnea (paras) should be eaten sitting on the threshold of the house and milk should be drunk with it; the woman who does this is bound to conceive.

4. Nine "tanks" of a combination of myrobalans, terminalia bellerica (beda) and hogplums, and one-and-a-quarter "tank" of arrowroot should be divided into three parts; each part should be taken on each day of the monthly course for three days and after it betel leaf prepared with betel nut, catechu, etc., should be eaten.

III

THE BATH FOR A WOMAN DESIROUS OF CHILDREN

Clay of a river bank and that of the bank of a rivulet, clay from seven wells, water of seven wells, clay of seven oil mills, dust of a place where three roads meet, the bark of plumbago zeylanica (chitra), yellow cotton pods, nine "tanks" of hogplums (ambala), the straws from the eaves of seven roofs of houses. All these should be collected and with these the barren woman should bathe naked under the eaves of the roof of the house and, bending the right foot, should offer handfuls of water to the Sun. After she has gone through this process, she should begin taking medicine.

IV

FOR HAVING REGULAR MENSES

1. By drinking a boiled decoction of mustard seeds, carrots (gajar) and date palm (suero) a woman gets regular monthly courses.

2. By crushing the seeds of the nimb and bambadoes aloes (sikotro), and keeping the lump near the mouth of the womb, a woman at once gets her menses.

3. The drinking of boiled decoction of solanum xanthocarpum (kshudra), the knot of bambadoes aloes (vanshi), sesamum (til), dill seeds (suva), bambadoes aloes (kunver) all taken in equal quantities and the application of the roots of euphorbia tirucalli (khardsani) to the mouth of the womb, a woman gets her menses at once.

V

FOR STOPPING MENSTRUATION

A pill made of blue vitriol (morthuthu), alum, aloes (aliyo), catechu, pamarix gallica (padvas) taken with sugar at the time of a woman's periods stops the menstruation.

VI

FOR PREVENTING CONCEPTION

A pill made of salt, alum, aloes (aliyo) and opium, all in equal proportion, placed in the mouth of the womb makes it hot, and this heat prevents conception.

VII

MATERIA MEDICA QUÆ IN ABORTIONE UTITUR

1. Kachi, id est aloes bambadosiensis, et aloes duo partes quindecim cum partibus olei calidi si bibit, conceptio omnino abit.

2. Mimasopis hexandræ, id est rajani semine, aloibus bambadosiensibus, id est sicotronc, necnon psitaccis, id est kuavæ, pluma applicatis abit stomachæ (*sic !*) perturoatio.

3. Pessa tam larga quam sagii, id est sodæ bicarbonatæ, grammum una cum arsenico, id est somalio, sale marino aloibusque applicata conceptio omnino abit.

4. Radicem nigodi, id est arboris castæ trifoliæ, una cum bœrhaviā verticillatā (kusudkhaprone) trituratam plumboque rubro (sinduro) in pessam fabricatam si in vagina retinet mulier medicina experta utetur mulier.

5. Pulsum (catholum), loranthum longiflorum (bandalum), aloes mimasopem hexandram (id est rajanum), sagonem (sabuchocam) boracem (tanchanum), sodam bicarbonatam (sajiam), turmericum, sal limumque æquis partibus triturata, et in pessam fabricata, si in vaginam inserit mulier, uteri perturbatione omnino obliviscit.

6. Plumbum, una cum nuce vomica (nepala) aloibusque æquis partibus combustum et bœrhaviæ diffusæ (id est satodinis) in radicibus trituratum medicamentum quam optimum præbet.

VIII

FOR INTESTINAL PAINS

1. The pain of the intestines (nal) will be removed by throwing three "tanks" of cyclea peltata (kadupad) in very hot clarified butter (ghee) made from cow's butter and by keeping a vessel of hot water on the belly.

2. The pain of the intestines (nal) is removed by eating asafœtida (hing), cumin seeds, coriander seeds, turmeric, orris root (pushkarmul) and plumbago zeylanica (chitramul), three kinds of salt and myrobalans, all in equal proportion.

IX

PAIN IN THE WAIST

1. Dry ginger, treacle and gum should be taken in equal proportion and clarified butter (ghee) equal to half the weight of them should be taken. Five "tanks" of this medicine taken daily remove the pain of the waist.

2. A pound of gruel made with clarified butter (ghee), treacle and gum should be mixed with simploces racemosa (lod), equal to four "pice" in weight, and the gum of odina nodier (baul) and paleteri root (akalkaro), each of the weight of two "pice" should be taken in the morning for pain in the waist.

X

RHEUMATISM OF THE WAIST

1. By drinking for seven days the fruits of coriander seeds or chiretta (kariyatu) pounded and mixed with castor oil the rheumatic pain of the waist is removed.

2. By drinking the flowers of the Indian lilace (nimb) tree, pounded in water, for seven days the pain in the stomach, the ribs, navel and the waist is removed.

3. Three "tanks" of cloves, dry ginger, pepper and black pepper (byosh), the outer shell of nutmeg (javantri), nutmeg, bay breng (vavading), paleteri root (akalkaro), cumin seeds (jeera), chiretta (kariyatu), cinnamon (taj), annamomum tomal (tamal), clerodendron serratum (bharang), the lesser galanjal (kulajon), pepper root, mesna ferrea (nagkeshar), three "tanks" should be pounded with three-quarters of a pound of treacle and pills should be made of them. By eating two "tanks" of these pills the stomach ache and rheumatism are cured.

END OF PART III

PART IV

INSANITY

Madness comes from offending the gods or the preceptor (guru); separation, evil spirits or irregular diet.

Characteristics

Fickleness of talent, absent-mindedness, laughter, excessive joy, shaking of the limbs, singing, dancing, weeping, stubbornness, cold limbs, restlessness and pain in neck, nose, ears, head, throat, teeth, anus, waist, navel, stomach, heart, secret parts, thighs and nails.

Remedy

Oils of three kinds should be well rubbed on the body and the body then be warmed.

For heavy breathing, weeping and mischief: turmeric, bilvoben (sanchal), asafœtida (ramath), dry ginger, white and black pepper (trikatu), and cumin seeds (jeera) should be powdered. Two "tanks" of this powder will cure the eighty-four kinds of diseases due to wind (vayu).

II

HARD BREATHING

1. Trichodesma Indicum (undhafali), brinjal (ringni), dry ginger, black and white pepper (trikatu), salt, bilvoben (sanchal), asafœtida, roots of castor oil plant (arand), common salt (kachlun) should be powdered in equal proportion and eaten with hot water to lessen hard, difficult breathing.

2. Good flowers of hellebore nigrum (kadu), pepper, cedar (sardaru) and dry ginger remove hard breathing.

3. If a man drinks the root of the flowering shrub (tagar), rubbed up into a paste with water, in whey for thirty-five days, not a trace of hard breathing will be left in his body.

Concoction—Quath

Adhatoda vasica (vasa), "jugirad-fali," tinospora cordifolia (akalkaro), taken in castor oil remove the pain of the stomach.

III

AM-VATA

1. Poor appetite, food can be taken in very small quantity, wind and passion in the body; these are the signs of (am-vata).

2. There is pain in the knees, waist, head and feet, cold and burning sensation in the body; these are the signs of (am-vata).

3. By drinking only four "tanks" of dry ginger with soup, (am-vata) and cough are cured.

4. Two "tanks" of castor seeds and one "tank" of myrobalans should be taken for seven days for curing (am-vata).

5. Piperchuba (chavyak), plumbago zeylanica (chitrak), dry ginger (nagar), and pepper longum (krishna) should be powdered and taken in hot water for curing this disease.

6. (am-vata) and pain in the waist are removed by drinking dry ginger, parsnip (ajmo), and padellium muracus (gokhru) boiled into a clear soup.

7. By eating curds, treacle, salt and butter, and avoiding the use of eatables that cause wind (vayu), in the body the am-vata is cured.

IV

DISEASES FROM

WIND (VATODAR), BILE (PITTODAR), AND PHELGM (KAFODAR)

When food is not well digested, and when there are no clear stools, wind, bile and phlegm are produced in the body.

Diagnosis

1. When there is pain in the stomach, and there is a noise in the stomach, it is due to wind (vatodar).

2. When there is burning sensation, giddiness, diarrhœa, and fever, it is due to bile (pittodar).

3. When there is hard breathing, thirst, sleeplessness, want of appetite, it is due to phlegm (kafodar).

4. When there is no liking for food and there is water in the stomach, it is dropsy (kathodar).

Medicines

1. Excess of phlegm (kafodar) is cured by drinking in water, salt, dry ginger, black and white pepper, parsnip and cumin seeds.

2. Excess of wind (vatodar) is cured by drinking salt and pepper with whey.

3. Excess of bile (pittodar) is cured by drinking pepper and sugar in water.

PAIN IN THE STOMACH

1. Residue of synapis alba (khol of sarasav) should be taken with whey for removing stomach ache.

2. Stomach ache is cured by pasting the stomach with the heated dung of a she-goat and antimony (sohiro).

3. Salt, aloes, salt-petre, the flour of millet, should be powdered and heated. These should be pasted on the stomach. After five days of this application, the pain in the stomach will vanish.

4. If a patient drinks powdered salt in whey for seven days, the pain in the stomach will vanish and cancer also will subside.

5. The seeds of the castor plant, bambadoes aloes (kachha) should be powdered and smeared on the belly for 3 days and heat (shek) be applied.

6. If a patient drinks three "tanks" of turmeric (rajani) and hornbeam-leaved cedar (balbeej) in clarified butter (ghee) in the morning, the pain in the stomach will vanish.

VI

LIMBS THAT ARE CRUSHED OR BEATEN

1. Turmeric and sugar should be eaten for internal effect; and, externally, for removing the pain of the limbs the leaves of the tamarind tree should be heated and tied on the limbs and warmth applied to them.

VII

HARD BREATHING WITH COUGH

1. If a child is given to drink only two grains of the concretions of the bile of an ox (ox-gall) rubbed in water, it will clear the belly and the cough will subside.

VIII

BURNING SENSATION

1. Copper sulphate (nilkanth), dry ginger, pepper, black cumin seeds (kalijeeri) should be powdered in water and smeared on the body, the patient will be free from all burning sensations in the body.
2. Burning sensation will be removed by smearing the body for seven days with all the five parts of leea robessta (kakjangha) powdered in water.

IX

MEDICINE FOR SKIN WRINKLED AND SPLIT ON ACCOUNT OF EXCESSIVE COLD

1. Litharge (mardarsingi), blue vitriol, resin, salt each weighing one "tank" and wax two "tanks," should be mixed with sixteen "tanks" of heated ghee. By applying this medicine to the wrinkled and split skin of the feet, the feet become soft.
2. Wax and ghee, two "tanks," and borax in weight half of them (i.e., one tank) should be heated and smeared on the feet, the pain from the cracks of the skin will be removed, and the skin will be soft.

X

CANCER OR BOIL

1. Salt, feronia elephantum (koth), sweet-flag root (vaj), pepper, orris root (pushkarmul), and turmeric should be powdered in water, and thickly smeared on the cancer or boil which will thereby subside.

2. Rondia dumeturum (mindal-arbud) and argemone Mexicana (chokh) should be rubbed in water and smeared on the cancer, which will subside and the pain will be removed.

XI

SKIN DISEASE CALLED KIDINAGARA

1. Nitrate of potash, blue vitriol, arsenic, lime, ashes of sesamum, dry stalks of " juvanbajri," carbonate of soda should be powdered in water in equal proportion and smeared on " kidinagara " for seven days.

2. The spot attacked with this disease should be washed with hot water, and then the powder of the Indian lilace (nimb) tree sprinkled on it; lime and carbonate of soda should then be applied on it.

3. Chimney smoke deposits, carbonate of soda, turmeric, lime, ashes of the peepal tree wood, should be powdered and a poultice be made of them and tied on the spot.

4. Pulse of roasted " math " seeds and blue vitriol; one fourth of this in weight should be powdered and mixed with the oil of synapis alba (sarasav) and applied on the spot.

XII

HOLES

1. Ashes of shell should be powdered in the juice of ark and then smeared on the hole with butter. The hole will be filled up.

XIII

SCROFULA

1. Synapis alba (sarasav), linseed, dill seeds, and tamarind should be mixed in whey and smeared on the throat.

2. Synapis alba (sarasav), and fruits of the babul tree should be burnt to ashes and blue vitriol should be taken in equal proportion and rubbed on the scrofulous part with mustard (sarasia) oil.

XIV

MEDICINE FOR PILES

1. Fruits of the Indian lilace (nimb) tree, and the oval-leaved rajabe should be powdered in equal proportion after baking them on the fire. That powder with sugar taken in the morning removes the piles.

2. Smoke of the horn of a cow should be given and fine powder of ivory and *troiling ecliptia (bhangaro)* should be crushed into a lump and tied on the piles. It will stop the bleeding of piles.

3. By eating two "tanks" of green turmeric with treacle in the morning for twenty-one days, the piles will vanish.

4. Seven "tanks" of butter, eight "tanks" of treacle, and seven "tanks" of elephant foot root (suran) should be taken for curing this disease.

XV

GIVING SMOKE TO THE PILES

1. Thorns of achjrontches aspera (agheda) equal to twenty "tanks" and five "tanks" of salt should be put on the fire and their smoke applied to the piles. This smoke should be given to the piles for twenty-one days, and during that time the man must abstain from eating saltish and sour substances. The piles will then subside.

2. The roots of plumbago zeylanica (chitra) should be rubbed in water and smeared on the piles; they will be dried up by this application.

3. Arsenic, argemone mexicana (chokh), alum, blue vitriol (morthuthu), lime and nitrate of potash should be pounded in the urine of a male and smeared on the piles for three days. They will be dried up by this application.

4. A poultice made of turmeric and ghee should be made and bandaged over the piles.

5. Blue vitriol and mercury should be pounded together and smeared on the piles for three days at night time. The piles will be cured.

6. Cyamojsis psoraloids (guvarsing) without seeds should be dried in the shade and powdered. This powder should be eaten for drying up the piles.

XVI

RED PILES

1. If a person eats eight "tanks" of butter and sesamum in the morning, red piles will subside. It is the best remedy.

2. Two "tanks" of the powder of elephant foot root (suran) should be mixed with curds and taken for seven days for removing red piles.

XVII

FOR BURNING SENSATION IN THE BODY

The body burns inwardly and outwardly; the belly remains heated; there is giddiness; these are the symptoms of the disease of burning sensation.

Remedies

1. Eaglewood (agar), cardemons, mild Himalaya cherries (padmak), sandalwood, cyrapus rotundas (moth) should be powdered and eaten with water.

2. Sandal and pepper should be powdered and sugar should be mixed with them. They should be taken with water for removing the burning sensation.

3. Ocymum basilicum (takmaria), cubeb pepper (kankol), kuskus grass (khas), sugar, and peppera longa should be kept soaked in water and two "tanks" of the water should be drunk at night. The body will have a cooling sensation.

4. Sulphur, purified in milk, should be pounded with the juice of potherb (cholai) and crystal and should be anointed on the body. It will cure the burning sensation.

5. A kind of fragrant root (kaempheria galangal) (kapurkachli), resin, costus root (kath), sandal, eaglewood and camphor should be pounded in equal proportion and smeared on the body. The pain will be removed.

6. Powder of resin, costus root (kath), cryapus rotundas (ghansar), eaglewood and mollotus philippinensis (kapilo) should be powdered in equal proportion and applied to the body.

7. If a person eats sulphur which is purified in milk with cumin seeds, the burning sensation in the body will be removed and his limbs will be good (sic.)

8. Fruits of the Indian lilace (nimb) tree, aniseed, sandal, eaglewood, cassia tora (punvad), catechu (kher), and oil prepared from resin should be eaten for curing the fever due to bile (pitt).

XVIII

MEDICINE FOR HEADACHE

1. Garlic, chiretta, pepper, and the outer shell of the coco-nut should be boiled, and that water drunk in the morning. The headache will be cured.

2. The root of conscura decussata (shankhavli) should be plucked on a Sunday morning, and after incense is applied to it, it should be kept on the head; the headache will be cured.

XIX

THE DROPPING OF THE NAVEL—PICHHOTI

If you can find the root of trianthema crystallina (punarnava-satodi) between the ruts of the wheels of a cart, you should pluck it on a Sunday. Having incensed it with bdellium (guggal), you should keep it in a small casket like a talisman, and you should bind that talisman on the waist for curing the dropping of the navel (pichhoti).

XX

STAMMERING—TREMBLE IN THE VOICE

If the voice is weak, or there is a tremble in the voice while speaking; if the limbs are discoloured and shake, there is stammering or trembling of the voice.

Remedies

1. Piper chaba (chavyak), dry ginger, ordinary pepper and black pepper, tamarind tree fruit, white cumin seeds, abies webbiana (talis), plumbago zeylanica (chitra), concretions of bile of an ox (gorochana), hogplums all in equal proportion should be powdered, and pills should be made of that powder with treacle, cardemons, cinnamon and cinnamomum tomal (tamal-patra). These pills will improve the voice.

2. If a person takes three "tanks" of pepper, terminalia bellerica (beda) and salt with cold water, his voice will improve.

3. Pepper, black pepper (mari), cardemons and salt should be powdered with treacle and drunk in cold water to improve the voice.

4. Two "tanks" of myrobalans (abhaya) should be drunk in water for seven days for improving the voice.

XXI

MEDICINE FOR EPILEPSY[1]

1. Dead locusts and ark (ankdo) should be ground in the juice of the latter. The powder thus prepared should be dried in the sunshine and again pounded. Pills as large as pepper should be made. These pills should be powdered, and the powder used like snuff at the time of the epileptic fit which will be stopped.

2. Barringtonia (samudrafal) should be pounded in the urine of a donkey and smelt every morning and evening for fourteen days. It will cure epilepsy.

3. Arsenic and a species of steatites (sankhjeera), one " tank " and one pound of the milk of a she-goat should be placed in an earthen pot, and the pot be placed in the midst of a heap of dung cakes and the whole fired. The medicine thus prepared should be taken equal in quantity to one " masa "[2] and pounded with the ghee of a cow. It should be taken for three days for curing epilepsy.

4. Tobacco, nuxvomica (jherkochla), the seeds of luffa achinata (kukadvela) and red chillies should be pounded in a mortar with the urine of an elephant for sixteen hours. At the time when the fit is on, a pipe of this medicine should be filled and the smoke imbibed—the fit will stop. Or if a person smells camphor and " kunkar " the fit will be over.

XXII

DYSENTERY OF CHILDREN—ATISAR

1. Holarrhena antidysenterica (kuda), turmeric of both kinds, licorice, pistacia integerrima (kakadsing), and the

[1] Number two was tried with remarkable success.—E. S.

[2] *See* Appendix B—Weights.

seeds of mangoes should be pounded in water and drunk for curing dysentery.

2. If a child is made to drink nutmeg and saxifraga ligulata (pakhan) rubbed over a stone in water, the passing of blood in diarrhœa or dysentery (atisar) will be stopped, and the body will become healthy.

3. Holarrhena antidysenterica (kuda), cumin seeds, greaslia tomentosa (dhavdi), sugar, gum of red silk cotton tree should be ground down in water, and that water should be drunk to prevent the passing of blood in dysentery (atisar).

4. Bell-tree fruit, cloves, aloes, greaslia tomentosa (dhavdi), peppera longa all in equal proportion should be powdered and mixed with honey and eaten during dysentery.

5. The blood passed in dysentery will stop flowing in the case of a child, if he be made to drink for four days continuously, dry ginger and saxifraga ligulata (bhed-pakhan) ground and mixed with water.

XXIII

MEDICINE FOR THE COLD OF A CHILD

1. Pistacia integerrima (kakadsing), cyrapus rotundas (moth), pepper, licorice all in equal proportion should be powdered, and a little licked in honey. This medicine will remove the cold.

2. Bell-tree fruit (bilva), aloes, greaslia tomentosa (dhavdi), parsnip (ajmo), all in equal proportion, should be powdered and drunk in water. This medicine will remove the pain in the stomach of a child.

3. Twenty "tanks" of pepper should be pounded in the juice of cactus and six pills should be given for removing stomach ache.

XXIV

MEDICINE FOR GETTING SLEEP

1. Pepper (white), musk (kasturi) . . . some words omitted . . . a man will at once get sleep and his body will become healthy.

2. Having procured the fruit of cytrus medica (matuling) put it on the head. The person thereby will fall so fast asleep that he will wake up only when he is called loudly.

XXV

BOILS (BAMLI) UNDER THE ARMPIT

1. The boils under the armpit will burst if salt and turmeric in bambadoes aloes (kumari) are bandaged over them.

2. Mollotus philippinensis (katilo), salt and turmeric powdered and applied remove the pain.

3. Bdellium (guggal), chimney smoke deposits (dhuso) and mustard, powdered and bandaged on the boils, will make them burst.

4. Lime, bark of pepper and salt should be heated and smeared over the boils.

XXVI

DELIRIUM OR PNEUMONIA

Symptoms

Fever, burning sensation, fatigue, red face, thirst, nervousness, diarrhœa, stained teeth and tongue are the symptoms of pneumonia.

Remedies

1. If a patient suffering from delirium is made to drink cumin seeds and a dead fly in cow dung, the disease will be cured.

2. Sandal, cardemons, cumin seeds and leaves of cumin seeds and leaves of ocymum sanctum (tulshi) should be pounded and given in water for curing delirium.

3. Cardemons, mild Himalaya cherries (padmak), cumin seeds, seeds of holarrhena antidysenterica (kuda) and purgative nut plant (nepala) should be pounded and drunk in water to cure delirium.

Decoction for Delirium

1. Sandal, cyrapus rotundas (moth), eaglewood, fumaria parviflora (purpat), green ginger, cinnamon tomal (tamalpatra) and chiretta (kariyatu) should be boiled together and drunk.

2. Sandal, small cumin seeds, cyrapus rotundas (moth), fumaria parviflora (papad), grapes, licorice (jethimadh), all should be boiled together and the decoction should be drunk with honey ; it cures delirium, fever, giddiness, etc.

XXVII

MAKING BLACK POWDER FOR TEETH[1]

A combination of myrobalans, terminalia bellerica (beda) and hogplums, gallnut, nutmeg, alum, catechu, cassia lancelata (sonamukhi), all in equal proportion, and the powder of simploces racemosus (lod) and coral (parwala) equal to it should be taken. These should be mixed with hogplums and juice of lemon and the juice of pomegranate twice as much. The powder mixed with all these

[1] Black teeth are fashionable amongst Mahomedan women, newly married.

juices should be dried, and after applying some sour substance to the teeth this powder should be rubbed over the teeth. By this the toothache will be cured, bad smell from the mouth will vanish, and the teeth will be cleaned.

XXVIII

RED POWDER FOR THE TEETH[1]

Skin of betel nut, catechu, crude sealing wax (lac) equal to seven "pice" in weight, Bengal mader roots (majith) should be pounded in water, and then crude sealing wax (lac) should be pounded with it; and a fine powder made. The powder should be dried in the shade and a sour substance should be rubbed on the teeth; this medicine should then be applied to the teeth when the teeth will be red.

[1] Red teeth are fashionable amongst Hindu newly married women. The translator saw some lovely sets of teeth ruined to look at by these fashions; but she is assured that teeth dealt with in this manner last their owner's lifetime and remain in good condition; and never ache.

END OF PART IV

PART V

POWDERS

(These powders are sold and are famous in India. They are called " Churna " and the recipes are kept very secret.)

POWDER OF CLOVES

Coco-nut, fruits of lotus, pepper, eaglewood (tagar), cubeb pepper, black cumin seeds, saffron, cloves, dry ginger, nutmeg, peppera longa, mesna ferrea, camphor, the white substance found in the bamboo, should be taken in equal proportion and powdered with sugar. This is lavingdi churna (powder of cloves) which cures gonorrhœa, peenus, hiccough and sore throat.

II

ASAFŒTIDA POWDER

Asafœtida, dry ginger, ordinary pepper and black pepper, myrobalans, deposits of smoke, parsnip, witchania sommi (asgandh), seeds of pomegranate, simploces racemosa (lod), nitrate of potash, orris root (pushkarmul), piper chaba (chavyak), cumin seeds, sandal, salt, plumbago zeylanica (chitra), sweet-flag root (vaj) should be powdered and "bhavana"[1] of the juice of citrus medica (bijora) should be given to them. This powder is called asafœtida powder and it cures cough, gulm and pain in the stomach.

III

GANGADHAR POWDER

Oval-leaved rajabe (indrajava), oroxylum Indicum (aralu), greaslia tomentosa (dhavdi), cyrapus rotundas (moth), dry ginger, parsnip, wild kuskus grass (padivalo), aconitum steterophyllum (ativakh), hellebore nigrum (kadu), simploces racemosa (lod), stone of a mango, gum of red silk cotton tree, cumin seeds, should be mixed with honey. This is gangadhar powder (churna) which cures dysentery (atisar) and makes a thin man fat.

ASAFŒTIDA (HINGASTAK) POWDER

Asafœtida, dry ginger, ordinary pepper and black pepper, parsnip (ajmo), salt and cumin seeds (ajmo). This is asafœtida (hingastak) powder which removes excess of wind and gives one a good appetite.

FOUR DRUGS WITH PLUMBAGO ZEYLANICA POWDER—CHITRACHOK POWDER

Myrobalans, salt, pepper, plumbago zeylanica (chitrak); all these four things should be powdered together in equal proportion. This powder will cure asthma, fever and cough.

[1] *See* Appendix A.

CARDEMONS POWDER

Cloves, cinnamomum tomal (tamal-patra), cardemons and mesna ferrea (nagkeshar), plumbago zeylanica (chitrak), dry ginger, ordinary pepper and black pepper, root of peppera longa, coriander seeds, bilvoben (sanchal), piper chaba (chavyak), parsnip (ajmo), winter cherries (asandh), sugar; all these should be powdered in equal proportion. This powder removes anæmia and cough.

TRISUGANDHADI POWDER

(The powder in which three well-flavoured drugs are the chief ingredients.)

Cloves, cinnamomum tomal (tamal-patra), cardemons, oriander seeds, tinospora cordifolia (galo), myrobalans (abhaya), terminalia bellerica (beda), and hogplums, bay breng (vavading), aniseed, dry ginger (sunth), peppera longa (krishna), turmeric, all the five parts of the bell-tree (bili), powder of rice and half the proportion of the ingredients of sugar. This powder is given for ring-worm, impurity of blood, anæmia and swelling due to excessive bile.

THE VICTORIOUS POWDER—VIJAYADI POWDER

Asafœtida, dry ginger, ordinary pepper and black pepper, weet-flag root (vaj), nitrate of potash, piper chaba (chavyak), two kinds of turmeric, bark of peepal tree, pulp of bell-tree fruit (bili), oval-leaved rajabe (indra-java), carbonate of soda, peppera longa of bigger type, castor oil tree root (arand), chiretta (kariyatu), parsnip (ajmo), five kinds of salt.[1] Two-and-a-half "tanks" of this powder should be taken at sunrise with hot water for the cure of asthma, swelling, anæmia, jaundice, gonorrhœa, sprue, fever and madness.

IV

THE POWDER OF SIXTEEN DRUGS—SHODSHANG POWDER

Cyrapus rotundas (moth), chiretta (kariyatu), hellebore nigrum (kadu), brinjal plant, dry ginger (sunth), pistacia integerrima (kakasing), orris root (pushkarmul), pepper root (kanak), pepper, trichosanthe cucumerina (patol), fumaria parviflora (purpat), coriander seeds (dhana), myrobalans (abhaya), cumin seeds, tinospora cordifolia (galo). This powder is given for slow fever, delirium and poverty of the vital fluids.

SHUDARSHAN POWDER

Dry ginger (sunth), ordinary pepper and black pepper, turmeric (rajani), berberis aristata (daruhaldar), solanum xanthocarpum (kshudra), cyrapus rotundas (moth), curcuma zedooria (sadi), tinospora cordifolia (galo), fumigatory (pitpapado), mild Himalaya cherries (padmak),

[1] *See* Appendix A—Note IV.

cassia occidentalis (kshundra), acinitum heterophyllum (ativakh), oval-leaved rajabe (indrajava), hellebore nigrum (kadu), hedy surumalhagi (dhamaso), kuskus grass (useer), plumbago zeylanica (chitro), parsnip (ajmo), cinnamon, bell-tree fruit (bili), red sandalwood, orris root (pushkarmul), trichosanthe cucumerina (patol), outer shell of nutmeg (javantry), bay breng (vadang), cedar (devdar), sweet-flag root (vaj), cloves (lavang), alum (turi), clerodendron serratum (bharangi), piper chaba (chavyak), chiretta (kariyatu), abies webbiana (talispatra) and parsnip (ajmo), bilvoben (sanchal), dry ginger (sunth) these three in equal proportion, and asafœtida, half of them, should be powdered. This powder removes excessive wind from the stomach and gives appetite.

END OF PART V

PART VI

PILLS

(These pills are, again, secret recipes in India.)

I

CAMPHOR PILLS

Camphor, a combination of myrobalans, terminalia (beda) and hogplums (trifala), nutmeg (jayfal), saffron (kesar), dry ginger (sunth), ordinary pepper and black pepper, cloves, paleteri root (akalkaro), the outer shell of nutmeg (javantry), bay breng of four kinds (vadang), gallnut adhatoda vasica (vasa), aconitum (vachhnag), clerodendron serratum (bharang), copper, catechu, nitrate of potash, dry ginger; all in equal proportion should be pounded in the juice of dry ginger (adrik). This pill should be taken in the juice of betel leaf. It cures asthma, weakness and gives good appetite.

II

BAY BRENG POWDER PILLS—VADANGANI PILLS

A combination of myrobalans, terminalia belletica (beda) and hogplums (trifala), dry ginger, ordinary pepper and black pepper, plumbago zeylanica (chitrak), bay breng (vadang) of four kinds, luffa achinata (jeemut), the white substance found in the bamboo (vanslochan), and snuff should be taken in ghee and honey in the morning. This cures gonorrhœa, anæmia, gulm and swelling.

III

CLOVE PILLS—LAVANGDI PILLS

A combination of myrobalans, terminalia bellerica and hogplums (trifala), cloves, cubeb pepper (kankol), cinnamon, cinnamomum tomal (tamal-patra), cardemons, mesna ferrea (nagkeshar), curcuma angustifolia (tabkhir), the white substance found in the bamboo (vanslochan), plumbago zeylanica (chitrak), and iron. All these should be powdered and taken with ghee and treacle in the morning. They cure swelling, rheumatism and jaundice (pandu).

IV

PILLS FOR WANT OF APPETITE—UNMILL

Myrobalans (abhaya-harade), dry ginger (sunth) and pepper should be pounded and pills made of them in treacle (gud). These pills cure want of appetite.

V

PILLS FOR CONSTIPATION

Salt, parsnip (ajmo), pepper, plumbago zeylanica (chitrak), bay breng (vidang), dry ginger (sunth), cedar, myrobalans (abhaya), dill seeds (suva), argyreia speciosa (bardha), and winter cherries (asandh). All these should be powdered and the powder be taken with treacle. It cures jaundice (pandu), constipation and want of appetite, and giddiness.

VI

ANANDBHAIRVA PILLS

Borax (tankankhar), pepper, aconitum (vachhnag), cloves, paleteri root (akalkaro), vermilion (sangrap), all in equal quantities, should be pounded in the juice of dry ginger (sunth) and pills made from them, two grams in weight. These pills should be given for delirium, cough, cold and windiness.

VII

CHINTAMANI PILLS

(The pills that give all wishes.)

Mercury (rasavisha), sulphur, borax (tankankhar), cumin seeds (jeera), mustard (rai), nitrate of potash (javkhar), a combination of dry ginger, ordinary pepper and black pepper, mica (abhrak), nitrate of potash (saji), aniseed (variyali), salt of five kinds ; all these should be pounded in the juice of lemon and ginger, and given in the leaves of the betel leaf. Cough, asthma, wind, indigestion of all kinds, delirium, peenus, blood coming from the mouth, leprosy, fistulas (bhagandars) and piles will be cured.

VIII

VADAVANAL PILLS

Lead, mercury (paro) and aconitum (vachhnag), each one " tank," salt, turmeric (haldar), nine " tanks " each, a combination of dry ginger, ordinary pepper and black pepper nine " tanks," plumbago zeylanica (chitrak) three " tanks " ; all these should be powdered. The powder should be mixed with cedar, ginger, citrus mediac (bijora) and juice of butea frondosa (khakhra) and smeared with the juice of the Indian lilace (nimb) tree and pepper; and given in betel leaf. These pills cure stomach ache, spasms of all kinds, gulm, catarrh, peenus, dyspepsia, want of appetite, giddiness and fever.

IX

YOGARAJ GUGGAL

Salt, plumbago zeylanica (chitrak), pepper, dill seeds (suva), casalpinia bonducella (kuver), cumin seeds (jeera), paleteri root (akalkaro), cedar (devdar), flour of gram, myrobalans, terminalia bellerica (beda) and hogplums (trifala), padellium muracus (gokhru), cyrapus rotundas (moth), piper chaba (chavyak), parsnip (ajmo), a combination of dry ginger, peppera longa and black pepper, kuskus grass (usheer), nutmeg (jayfal), cinnamon (taj), cinnamomum tomal (tamal-patra), sweet-flag root (vaj), cardemons, costus root (kuth), mesna ferrea (nagkeshar), bay breng (vading) should all be taken in equal quantities and pounded, and twice as much good bdellium as that powder should be pounded with it. Pills made of this powder cure windiness (vayus) of all kinds, stimulate the appetite, cure worms, itch and shooting pains.

AGASTYA PILLS—No. 1

Sulphur, cenabar (hingalo), one "tank" each; two "tanks" of opium, half a "tank" of aconitum (vachhnag), cumin seeds (jeera) and nutmeg six "tanks." These pills are given for windiness, swelling, cough and shooting pains.

XI

ANANDBHAIRVA PILLS

Anandbhairva pills of sulphur (gandhak) and mercury (paro) in equal weight, and purgative nut plant equal to the weight of both, myrobalans, terminalia bellerica (beda) and hogplums (trifala) should be taken with betel leaf to cure fevers of all kinds.

XII

AGASTYA PILLS—No. 2

Ten "tanks" of nuxvomica (jherkochla) should be boiled and then passed through a thin cloth. Th following medicines, each two "tanks" in weight, should be mixed with it: Casalpinia bonducella (kuber), dry ginger (sunth), long pepper and black pepper, paleteri root (akalkaro), asafœtida (hing), bay breng (bidang), mercury (rasa), sulphur (gandhak), and cubeb pepper (kankol). The pills made of these cure wind (vayu), gulm, worms, swelling, dyspepsia, cold and gonorrhœa.

END OF PART VI

PART VII

OINTMENTS

GHRITA—MEDICINAL GHEES

(In India these ointments are eaten.)

Cyrapus rotundas (moth), chiretta (kariyatu), oval-leaved rajabe (indrajava), Indian lilace (nimb) tree fruit, trianthema crystallina (purva), tinospora cordifolia (galo), asparagus racemosus (satvari), costus root (kuth), citrusllus colocynthus (indrani), fumigatory (pitpapdo), hemidesmus Indicus (sariva), berberis aristata (daruhaldar), licorice (jethimadh), purging cassia (girmalo), aconitum heterophyllum (ativish), adhatoda vasica (ardushi), mild Himalaya cherries (padmak), curcuma zedoória (sadhi), pepper, black hemidesmus Indicus (black sariva), cyclea peltata (padi), turmeric (nisha), sweet-flag root (vaj), hogplums (ambala), bark of caledupa arborea (karanj), valesiana wallichii (tagar), seeds of lotus, nutmeg, elephant foot root (suran)—not much grown—herpestis momnaiera (brahmi), roots of alhagi maurorum (javasimul), mesna ferrea (nagkeshar), greaslia tomentosa (dhav-chopdo) should be taken in equal weight.

All together eight pounds of these should be boiled in one "drona"[1] (1,024 tolas) of water. Half a maund of the juice of hogplums (ambala), two pounds of ghee and the above-mentioned medicines should be boiled together and the ghee left behind should be taken up carefully. This ghee cures leprosy, delirium, boils, scrofula, worms (gajcharam).

[1] *See* Appendix B—Weights.

II

BRAHMI GHRITA

Herpestis momnaiera (brahmi), sweet-flag root (vaj), conscura decussata (sankhavli), myrobalans, terminalia bellerica (beda) and hogplums (trifala), root of cephalandra Indica (dodimul), pomegranate, costus root (kuth), pepper, cyrapus rotundas (moth), kuskus grass (useer), padellium muracus (gokhru), cyclea peltata (pad), cardemons, white substance found in the bamboo (vanslochan), ficus Bengalensia (vad), powder of dates, adhatoda vasica (vasa), sugar, dry ginger, cumin seeds, ocymum sanctum (tulshi), desmadium gangeticum (salivani), leaves of jasmanium (jai), orris root (pushkarmul), cedar (devdar), ghee; and milk four times the weight of these medicines; should, all of them, be boiled on a slow fire. The ghee left behind should be used as a specific for curing madness, and weakness of intellect.

III

BENGAL MADER ROOT GHRIT—MAJITHDI GHRIT

Bengal mader roots (majith), turmeric (nisha), hellebore nigrum (kadu), aconitum heterophyllum (ativakh), cedar (devdar), dry ginger (sunth), sweet-flag root (vaj), myrobalans (abhaya), parsnip (ajmo), asafœtida, all these should be boiled in one pound of water. When less than one pound of water has been left behind, the ghee can be used for hiccough, asthma, gonorrhœa, sprue, cough and indigestion.

IV

GARLIC MEDICINAL GHEE—LASAN GHRIT

Garlic, alhagi mourorum (javasa), brinjal plant, each two pounds, should be boiled in one "drona"[1] of water and when one-fourth of the water is left behind, it should be taken down from the fire. Half a maund of raisins, two pounds of ghee and milk, lemon, pepper one "pal," ceropegia bulbosa (kudher) three "pals,"[1] and the juice of adhatoda vasica (vasa) should be mixed with them, and they should be placed on a slow fire. A quarter of a pound of sugar and oil, half a pound of honey, five "tanks" of tobacco should be added. This ghee cures slow fever, jaundice and consumption.

THE GHEE OF THE THREE FRUITS—TRIFALA GHRITA

The juice of a combination of myrobalans terminalia bellerica (beda) and hogplums (trifala), and adhatoda vasica, each one pound in weight, should be boiled in one pound of milk and two pounds of ghee. The following medicines in equal quantities should then be mixed with them: "Kanklata," cubeb pepper (kankol), salt, seeds of lotus, licorice (jethimadh), dry ginger (sunth), pepper, turmeric, sugar and boerhavia diffusa (satodi). This ghee cures itch and scurvy.

[1] *See* Appendix B—Weights.

VI

THE GHEE OF THE GODDESS OF LEARNING—SARASVATI GHRITA

Eight pounds of the juice of jasmanium (brahmi), two pounds of honey and ghee, turbeeth root (nisot), turmeric (nisha), myrobalans (abhaya) one "pal"; adhatoda vasica (vasa), salt, pepper, sugar, bay breng (vading) each two "tanks" and a half in weight should be boiled in eight pounds of water. When one-fourth of the water is left behind, this ghee and juice should again be boiled. The ghee left behind should then be taken out and used for deafness. It increases brain-powder and sharpens the memory to such an extent that that which is read or memorised to-day will be remembered, at least, for a month. This is called Sarasvati ghrita.

VII

THE GREAT GHEE—MAHAGHRITA

The fruits of the Indian lilace (nimb) tree, cyrapus rotundas (moth), chiretta (kariyatu), aconitum heterophyllum (ativish), a combination of myrobalans, terminalia bellerica (beda) and hogplums (trifala), pepper, hellebore nigrum (kadu), sweet-flag root (vaj), adhatoda vasica (vasa), turmeric, trichosanthe (kadu), fumigatory (pitpapdo), tinospora cordifolia (galo), hemidesmus Indicus (sariva), the fruit pulp of the purging cassia (girmalo), alhagi mourorum (javaso), licorice (jethimadh), costus root (kuth); all these should be pounded and boiled in eight times their weight in water. Four pounds of the juice of hogplums (ambala), two pounds of cows' ghee should then be boiled with them. The ghee left behind should be taken and used in the cure of scrofula, hemorrhages, boils, pimples and leprosy.

VIII

THE PEACEFUL GHEE—KALYAN GHRITA

Abies webbiana (talish), a combination of myrobalans, terminalia bellerica (beda) and hogplums (trifala), aloes (aliyo), sandal, pomegranate, turmeric of both kinds, sweet-flag root (vaj), cloves, cinnamon cedar (devdar), desmadium gangeticum (salivani), hemidesmus Indicus (sariva), Bengal madder roots (majith), mild Himalaya cherries (padmak), costus root (kuth), the seeds of the lotus, asafœtida, eaglewood (tagar), bay breng (vadang), garlic, cardemons, all should be taken in equal proportion. All of them should weigh one pound and they should be boiled in four times as much water and ghee. The ghee that is left behind is Kalyan ghrita.

END OF PART VII

PART VIII

OILS

ASPARAGOPSIS RACEMOSUS—SATAVARI OIL

Two seers[1] of the juice of asparagopsis racemosus (satavari), should be mixed with one seer each of the milk of the cow and the buffalo. Then winter cherries (asandh), boerhavia diffusa (satodi), asafœtida, each one "pal" in weight should be pounded and passed through a thick cloth. These medicines together with the two pounds of oil already boiled should be reboiled with the following medicines: Costus root (kuth), turmeric, acacia catechu (kher), berberis aristata (daru-haldar), bay breng (vadang), nitrate of potash (javkhar), pepper, dry ginger, licorice (jethimadh) all powdered. The oil which is left after this boiling is the asparagopsis racemosus (satavari) oil first invented by Muni Waghji and this oil cures all windiness.

II

KUSHTADI OIL

Cropegia acuminata (girtumbi), costus root (kuth), licorice (jethimadh), cedar (devdar), dry ginger (sunth),

[1] *See* Appendix B—Weights.

long pepper and black pepper, bambadoes aloes (kunver), argemone Mexicana (chokh), sweet-flag root (vaj); all these should be taken in equal proportion—but all together in weight only sixteen "vals"[1]—and eighteen "tanks" of oil mixed with them. This oil is called "kushtadi" oil and gives great ease to the body when it is rubbed with it. It also cures all diseases of the head.

III

GIGANTIC SOLVERT OIL—ARK OIL

The juice of the gigantic solvert (ark) and thorn apple (dhaturo) plant and the urine of a cow equal in weight to one "pal,"[1] two "pals" of the roots of the castor oil plant (arand), and eight "pals" of oil, mardostachys jatamanse (badabavil), sandal, sweet-flag root (vaj), cedar (devdar), costus root (uplot), dry ginger (sunth) should all be powdered and boiled in oil. This oil cures that disease in which the limbs of the body shake perpetually.

IV

MYROBALANS OIL—HARADIS OIL

Yellow orpiment (harital), turmeric, realgar (mansil). a combination of myrobalans, terminalia bellerica (beda) and hogplums (trifala), alum, Bengal mader roots (majith), iron sulphate (kashis), and sulphur (gandhak) should be boiled in oil in a big copper saucepan. This oil will cure the itch.

[1] *See* Appendix B—Weights.

V

SULPHUR OIL—GANDHAK OIL

Yellow orpiment (harital), sulphur, realgar (mansil), plumbago zeylanica (chitrak), pepper, red lead (sindur), mollotus philippinensis (kapilo), carbonate of soda (saji), asculint flacursia (bawachi), cassia tora (puvad), alum (turi), and borax (tankankhar) should all be boiled in the oil of globra (karanj) and the ghee of the cow. This oil cures itch.

VI

THE VICTORIOUS GOD'S OIL—VIJAYABHAIRAVA OIL

Mercury (rasa), sulphur (gandhak), yellow orpiment (hari), realgar (mansil) should be powdered and bound in a cloth. They should then be burnt[1] over a lamp of oil under which a vessel is placed to collect the oil which falls from the lamp. This oil cures the trembling of the limbs of the body.

VII

NARAYAN OIL

Bell-tree root (bili), clerodendron phlomoides (arani), brinjal, oroxylum Indicum (arlu), sterio spermum chelonoides (padalmul), winter cherries (aswagandh), abutilon Indicum (atibal), padellium muracus (gokhru), two-and-a-half " tanks " all in equal proportion; six maunds of the juice of asparagopsis racemosus (satavari), one maund of

[1] This to me appears dangerous.

oil and eighteen maunds of water should be boiled together. The oil that is left behind should be mixed with cedar (devdar), herpestis momnaiera (brahmi), dill seeds (suva), garlic, cardemons, eaglewood (tagar), cloves, boerhavia diffusa (satodi) and cyrapus rotundas (kuth); all in equal proportion should be thrown in that oil, and this oil when rubbed on the body cures rheumatism.

APPENDIX A

GAJPUTMUDRA

The "Gajput" process requires the construction of a pit in the ground two feet by two feet square, and two feet deep. In this pit dry cow-dung cakes collected in their natural state from the jungle should be put, and then fire set to them; the medicine which must be put in vessels in the pit should be kept burning till the dung-cakes burn out and the medicine is quite cool.

"Mudra": Two vessels with their mouths bound to each other so firmly as to preclude all possibility of the air getting in are called "Mudra." The medicine to be treated is contained in the "Mudra."

II

PUTPAK

Any medicinal powder or mixture should be well covered up between layers of the leaves of the castor oil plant, or of the Jambu tree; and over this a layer of earth an inch thick should be put. After the earth dries, it should be baked red hot over a fire. It should, then, be taken out of the fire and the earth removed.

The juice that is thus formed should be strained; and this is called "putpak."

III

BHAVANA

Any powdered drug when fully mixed with the juice of some other drug and the mixture thus made thoroughly ground in a pestle and mortar until it becomes very fine is called Bhavana.

IV

Five kinds of salt :—

1. Sindhalun, rock salt (reddish) ;
2. Sanchal (bilvoben), black salt ;
3. Bid-lun ;
4. Vadagaru salt ; and
5. Salt obtained from the sea.

The other salts are Potashes and Sodas.

APPENDIX B

WEIGHTS

One tank is equal to half a tola.
One pal is equal to 2 tolas.
One masa is equal to 12 grains.
One val is equal to 6 grains.
One chanothi is equal to 2 grains.
One gunja is equal to 2 grains.
One drona is equal to 1,024 tolas.
A seer is one pound in Kathiawar, two pounds in Bengal, and in liquid weight a pint.

INDEX

(Indian name in brackets and indication of the drug's use.)

Abies Webbiana (talispatra)—Stammering.

Accacia Catechu { kadvi, khadir, kher } Pain in the ear; gonorrhœa; ecthyma.

Achjrontches aspera { agadi, agheda } Syphilis; boils; ulcers; piles.

Aconitum (vachhnag)—Poisoning.

Aconitum heterophyllum { ativasa, ativakh } Dysentery.

Acorus calamus (vaj)—Delirium.

Adhatoda vasica { ardushi, vasa, vasu } Delirium; jaundice; nose-bleeding tooth-ache; gonorrhœa.

Adiantum lunulatum (hanspadi)—Carbuncle; gonorrhœa.

Alhagi mourorum root { javaso, javasimul } Pain in the vagina.

Aloes (jeera)—Ecthyma; diarrhœa.

Aloewood (agar)—Bad smell in the vagina.

Alum { fatakdi, turi } Piles; tooth-ache, hair dye; burning sensations in vagina.

Ani seeds (variyali)—Burning sensation in vagina; other burning sensations.

Antimony (sarma)—Nose-bleeding; gonorrhœa.

Argemone maxicana (chokh)—Ecthyma; piles.

Arsenic (somal)—Consumption; piles.

Asculint flacursia { babachi, bavchi } Itch; blood-poisoning or tiger. mauling; wounds; loss of vital fluids.

Asparagopsis racemosus (satvari)—Gonorrhœa.
Asparagus ascendens (musali)—Gonorrhœa; loss of vital fluids.
Assafœtida { rath / ramath } Delirium; worms; guinea worms; blood-poisoning.

B

Bambadoes aloes { kunver / koover } Stomach-ache; piles; cough of consumption; for retentive power.
Bamboo (bas)—Jaundice; urethra stricture; leuccorrhœa.
Barberis aristata (darunisha)—Jaundice.
Barley (java)—Diarrhœa.
Barringtonia (samudrafal)—Epilepsy.
Bay breng { bidang / vidang } Stomach-ache; blood-poisoning; tiger mauling.
" " (vavading)—Cold; partial headache.
Bdellium (guggal)—Swelling; syphilis; boils; ulcers; wounds; cough of consumption.
Bell-tree fruit (beel)—Delirium; diarrhœa; dysentery.
" " (bilva)—Syphilis; boils; ulcers.
" root (biljada)—Delirium.
" juice (bilisara)—Diarrhœa; dysentery.
" powder (biluchur)—Dysentery.
Bengal maderroots (majith)—Delirium; leucorrhœa; tooth-ache; gonorrhœa; wounds.
Benicassa cerifera (gir)—Poisoning.
Berberis aristata { daruhaldar / rasvanti } Nose-fistula; wounds.
Betel nut (sopari)—Stomach-ache; syphilis; boils; ulcers.
Bilvoben (sanchal)—Diarrhœa; stomach-ache; worms; ear-ache; leprosy.
Boerhavia diffusa { satodi / Punarnava } Gonorrhœa.
Boerhavia verticillach (pat khapariyo)—Nose-bleeding.
Borax { tankhankhar / tankhan } Piles; consumption; tooth-ache; poison of snake.

Cactus (thor)—Syphilis; boils; ulcers; stomach-ache; piles; tooth-ache.
Calcium sulphate (godanta)—Ecythma; piles; consumption; gonorrhœa.
Caledupa arborea (karanj)—Syphilis; boils; ulcers.
Camel thorn (javas)—Urethra stricture.
Camphor (kapur)—Cold; ecthyma; piles; epilepsy.
Cannabis sativa (bhang)—Itch; guinea worm.
Cappasis aphylla (kerada)—Nose-fistula.
Carbonate of soda { sajikhar / sachro } Ear-ache; piles; scrofula.
Cardemous (alachi)—Cold; nose bleeding; bad smell in the mouth; gonorrhœa; stammering.
Casalpinia bonducella { kuber / kuver } Stomach-ache; cough of consumption.
" " (kankachi)—Leucorrhœa.
Cassia lanceolata (sonamukhi)—
Cassia occidentalis (kshundra)—Worms.
Cassia toa (puvad)—Babhuti.
Castor plant (arand)—Diarrhœa; dysentery; burns.
Catechu { katho / kher } Syphilis; boils; ulcers; tooth-ache; burning sensations.
Cedar (devdar)—Tongue diseases; diarrhœa; jaundice; dysentery; cold; swelling; ecthyma; gonorrhœa.
" (balbeej)—Leucorrhœa.
Cenabar (hingalo)—Pain in the ear.
Cephalondra Indica (tindori)—Pain in the ear.
Cherries, mild Himalaya (padmak)—Wounds.
China root (chop chini)—Loss of vital fluids.
Chiretta { kariatu / bhunimb } Profuse menstruation; delirium; tongue disease; stomach-ache; headache.
Christmas rose (katuk)—Delirium; tongue disease; diarrhœa; dysentery; jaundice.
Cida carpinifolia (gangeru)—
Cida spinosa (nagbala)—
Citrus colocynthis { trush / indrani } Stomach-ache.

Citrus medica { matuling / bijora } Colic.

Clarified butter (ghee)—Jaundice; poisoning; ecthyma; carbuncle; burns; leucorrhœa; syphilis; tooth-ache; nose-fistula; poison of snake.

Clematir (murva)—

Clerodendron phlomoids (arno)—Pain in the ear; swelling.

Clerodendron serrotum (bharangi)—Tongue disease.

Cloves (lavang)—Cold; nose-fistula; loss of vital fluids; diarrhœa.

Colocynth (indravarna)—Cough of consumption; impotency.

Concretions of bile of an ox (gorochana)—

Conscura decussàta { funidadi / sankhavli / chadgan } Piles; headache.

Copper sulphate (nilkanth)—Burning sensations.

Corchorus antichorus (bahufali)—Leucorrhœa.

Cordia latifolia (gundi)—Syphilis; ulcers.

Coriander seeds (sokh)—Diarrhœa; cold; poison; dysentery; leucorrhœa.

Costus root (kath)—Syphilis.

(kauth)—Diarrhœa; jaundice; worms; burns; burning sensations.

(kuthvadi)—Dysentery; leprosy.

(uplot)—Wounds.

Croton triglium (dati)—Stomach-ache.

Cubeb pepper (kankol)—

Cubebs (kababchini)—

Cumin seeds { jeera / jirak } Diarrhœa; dysentery; nose-bleeding; leucorrhœa; gonorrhœa; stammering.

Curcuma zedooria { sadhai / sadhi } Worms; tongue disease; delirium; dysentery.

Cyamojsis psoraloids (guvar)—

Cyclea peltata (padh)—Tongue disease; delirium.

Cynodon ductylon { dhro / dhruva } Nose-bleeding.

Cyperus hexastachyus (nagermoth)—

Cyrapus rotundas	ghausar moth	Delirium; tongue diseases; jaundice; dysentery; worms; ear-ache; swelling; blood-poisoning or tiger mauling; burning sensations.

Cytrus (amalvetus)—Dysentery.
(bijora)—Tongue diseases; ear-ache.
Cytrus medica (bijora)—Pain in the ear.

Dandelion (dudheli)—Impotency; leucorrhœa.
Delirium (bhagna netra)—
Deposits of smoke (dhuso)—
Desmodium gangeticum (salavani)—Dysentery.
Dill seeds (suva)—Delirium; diarrhœa; stomach-ache; dysentery; pain in the ear.
Dry ginger—Pepper (ordinary).
Peppera longa (vyokh)—Cold.

Dry ginger	sunth nagar	Tongue diseases; delirium; diarrhœa; cold; jaundice; dysentery; hiccough; swelling; pain in the vagina; pimples on the face; excessive menstruation; loss of vital fluids; stammering.

Eaglewood	tagar krishnagar maliageru	Delirium; burning sensations.

Echinatus (utkanto)—Retentive power.

Fat (charmi)—
Fenel seeds (shauff)—Jaundice.

Feronia elephantum { koth / kauth } Hair dye; nose-bleeding; leucorrhœa; gonorrhœa.
Ferri sulphate (geru)—Syphilis; boils.
Ferri sulphate, natural (shankhgeru)—Gonorrhœa.
Ficus Bengalensia (vad)—Impotency.
Ficus glomerata (umber)—Impotency.
Fœungreek grass (methi)—Tooth-ache.
Fogonia Arabica { dhana / vavasakh } Profuse menstruation.
Fragrant root (papurkachli)—
Froma elephantum (koth)—Diarrhœa; dysentery.
Fumaria parviflora (purpat)—
Fumaria periflora (papad)—
Fumigatory (pitpapdo)—Profuse menstruation.

Gallnut (maju)—Tooth-ache.
{ maya / mayafal } Pain in the ear; piles; syphilis; boils; gonorrhœa.
Garlic (lasan)—Delirium; guinea worms; headache.
Gassypium arboreum (hirdhan)—Poison.
Gigantic solvert (ankdo)—Pain in the ear; cough of consumption; blood poisoning; whitlow; tiger mauling; epilepsy.
Glycyrrhisa glabara (madhurmuli)—
Grapes (drokh)—Delirium.
Greaslia tomentosa (dhavdi)—Diarrhœa; dysentery; leucorrhœa.
Gum of red silk cotton tree (mochrasa)—Diarrhœa.
Gymnema sylvestres (massringi)—
Gymnosparia montana (vikaj)—Wounds.

H

Hedysurum alhagi (dhamaso)—Tongue diseases.
Hellebore nigrum { kadu / rohini } Swelling; tooth-ache.
Herpestis momnaiera (bahmi)—Tongue diseases.

Hogplums (ambala)—Gonorrhœa; cold; jaundice; piles; wounds.
Holarrhena antidysenterica (kuda)—Diarrhœa; dysentery.
Honey (madhu)—Jaundice.
Hornbeam-leaved cedar (bal)—Delirium.
Horseradish tree (saradhu)—Jaundice; pain in the ear.
Hygrophila spinosa (akhro)—Leucorrhœa; gonorrhœa; loss of vital fluids.
Hemidesmus Indicus (sariva)—Wounds.
Henbane (khurasan)—Retentive power.

I

Indian jalup (nishot)—Piles.
Indian mazorian (girani)—Pain in the ear.
Indian mello (kangsa)—Cold; boils; dysentery.
Indian plimywort (brahmi)—

Jasmanium (jai)—
Jasminum grandiflorum (chambeli)—Leprosy; retentive power. (Jasmine)

K

Kaempferia galangal (kapurkachli)—
Khuskhus grass — chalak, valo, khas, lochan — Dysentery; whitlow; bad smell in the vagina.

Lac (lakh)—Babuti; leucorrhœa.
Lawsonia inermis (mendi)—Carbuncle.
Leea robessta (kakjungha)—Piles.
Licorice (jethimadh)—Diarrhœa; hiccough; cold; impotency; stricture of the urethra; burning sensations in the vagina; gonorrhœa.

Lilace fruit (Indian-nimb)—Burning sensations.
Lime (chunam)—Piles; bite of rabid dog.
Linseed (alsi)—
Litharge { bodar / murdasingi } Syphilis; ulcers.
Lorangthus longiflorus (bandal)—
Lotus { kaj / kamalkakdi } Lotus seeds.
(kamal)—Cold.
Lotus bulb (kaselo)—Syphilis; boils; ulcers.
Louse (guti)—
Luffa achinata (bindali)—Peenus.
(kukadvala)—Epilepsy.

M

Macuna pruriens (kavuch)—
(madki)
Madder-roots—Bengal-majith.
Mango (amb)—
Marking nuts (bhilama)—
Mercuras sulphide (kajali)—Ecthyma.
Mercury (ras)—Itch; piles.
Mercury and sulphur (kajeli)—Syphilis; boils; ulcers.
Mesna ferrea (nagkeshar)—Gonorrhœa; diarrhœa; dysentery; leucorrhœa; bad smell in the mouth.
Mimsoaps hexandra (ryan)—
Mimosa catechu (kher)—Worms.
Mollotus philippinensis (kapilo)—Syphilis; ulcers; boils; burning sensations.
Mustard (rai)—
Mustard pod (raising)—Guinea worms; carbuncle.
Myrobalans (abhaya)—Diarrhœa; itch; jaundice; dysentery and stammering.
Myrobalans harade / harada — Pain in the stomach; swelling; burns; peenus; piles; gonorrhœa; wounds; stammering; worms.
Mysore gambostree (revanchi)—Poisoning of rabid dog and mad fox.

N

Natural ferri sulphate (geru)—Poison of rabid dog or fox.

Nimb (nimb tree). (The Indian lilace tree.) Jaundice; bad smell in the vagina; piles; leprosy; blood-poisoning or tiger mauling.

Nitrate of potash (javakhar)—Delirium; stricture of the urethra; leprosy.

Nitron (sajikhar)—Pain in the stomach.

Nutmeg { jatifal / jayafal } Bad smell in the mouth; loss of vital fluids; impotency.

Nutmeg, outer shell (javantri)—Loss of vital fluids; retentive power.

Nuxvomica (jherkochla)—Poisoning.

O

Ocymum sanctum (tulsi)—Hiccough; stomach-ache.

Ocymum sanctum, black—Loss of vital fluids.

Odina nodier gum (bol)—

Oleander, sweet-scented (kaner)—

Opium (safain)—Guinea worms; retentive power.

Orchis latifolia (salam)—Loss of vital fluids.

Oroxylum Indicum (arlu)—

Orris root (pushkarmul)—Tongue disease; worms; delirium.

Oval-leaved rajabe (indrajava)—Diarrhœa; dysentery; worms; piles; ecthyma.

Ox-gall (rochana)—Gonorrhœa.

Paddy seeds (lazakhan)—Cold.

Padellium muracus (gokhru)—Diarrhœa; dysentery; stricture of the urethra; gonorrhœa; loss of vital fluids.

Paleteri root { akalkaro / marhatti } Piles; loss of vital fluids; retentive power.

Pandanus foscicularis (ketaki)—Retentive power.

Pandonus adoratissimus (kevada)—Hair dye.

Parsnips (ajmo)—Diarrhœa; stomach-ache; dysentery.
(javani)—Tooth-ache; gonorrhœa.

Pepper peepli kana — Delirium; diarrhœa; hiccough; peenus; tooth-ache; nose fistula; excessive menstruation; headache; stammering.

Pepper root (granthik)—Diarrhœa; jaundice; colic; dysentery.

Persian lilac (bakayani)—

Piper chaba (chavyak)—Stammering.

Piper cubeb (shitalchini)—Loss of vital fluids.

Pistachia integerrima (kaksingi)—Tongue diseases; jaundice; worms; cough of consumption; diarrhœa.

Plumbago zeylanica (chitra)—Swelling; ecthyma; delirium; stammering; diarrhœa; dysentery; piles.

Pongunia globra (karanja)—Piles; wounds.

Poparlind figtree { piparo pipalo } Syphilis; boils; ulcers.

Poppy (posat)—Ecthyma.

Poppy seeds (khuskhus)—Burns; loss of vital fluids.

Pot-herb { cholai tandaljo } Poison of serpent; leucorrhœa.

Prickly plant (dhamaso)—Tongue disease; stomach-ache; guinea worms.

Pumpkin (kola)—Poisoning.

Purple goat's rue (sarpankho)—Ecthyma.

Pudding pipe-tree (girmalo)—Delirium; gonorrhœa.

Purgative nut plant nepala ajepal — Poisoning; stomach-ache; ecthyma; piles.

Purging cassia pulp gir girmalo — Poisoning; pain in the stomach; stricture of the urethra; gonorrhœa.

Quercus infectorius mayafal manjfal mangfal — Piles.

Radish (muli)—Babuti.
Rajabe, oval-leaved (Indajava)—
Randia dumeturum { mainal / mindalarbud } Poisoning.
Rasa (mercury)—Itch.
Realgar (mansil)—Partial headache; ecthyma; cough of consumption; wounds.
Red lead (sindhur)—Syphilis; boils; ulcers; wounds; impotency.
Red ochre (geru)—Nose fistula.
Red silk cotton tree (mochrasa)—Dysentery.
Resin { ral / saramras } Dysentery; nose-bleeding; burning sensations; piles.
Roots, ten roots combination (deshmul)—Delirium.
Rose (shatpatra)—Cold.
Rose apple (ramfal)—

Saffron (keshar)—Retentive power.
Saffron wild (kasumbi)—Loss of vital fluids.
Salt (sindhav)—Itch; cold; guinea worms; stammering.
Salt mineral (sindhalun)—
Saltishearth (khara)—Piles.
Sandal wood (sukhad)—Cold; leucorrhœa; colic; burning sensations.
Sandal wood, red (ratanjali)—Nose fistula; wounds.
Saxifraga ligulata { bhed / pakhan } Diarrhœa; stricture of the urethra.
Scirpus kysoor (kasel)—Leucorrhœa.
Senna (sonamukhi)—Poisoning; leucorrhœa.
Sesamum oil—Poisoning.
Shells (chip)—Leprosy.
Simploces racemosa (lod)—Diarrhœa; dysentery; worms; tooth-ache; wounds.
Soapnut, country (aritha)—Partial headache; tooth-ache.
Solanum jacquinum (bhorangi)—Worms.
Solanum xanthocarpum (kshundra)—Tongue diseases; ecthyma; cough of consumption.

Spykenard valeriana (tagar)—Loss of vital fluids.

Staff tree { kangni / mal-kangni } Loss of vital fluids.

Steatities species (shankhjeera)—Epilepsy.

Sugar (sita)—Diarrhœa; jaundice; dysentery; hiccough; gonorrhœa.

Sulphate of mercury (hingalo)—Ecthyma.

Sulphur { gandhak / amalsar } Itch; ecthyma; burning sensations.

Synapis alba { sarasav / katu } Jaundice; itch; pain in the ear; partial headache; scrofula.

Sweet-flag root (vaj)—Diarrhœa; dysentery; worms; pain in the ear; partial headache; pimples of the face.

Sweet-scented oleander (kaner)—Retentive power.

Tamarix gallica (padvas)—

Terminalia bellerica (beda)—Cold; poisoning; swelling; peenus; leucorrhœa; piles; gonorrhœa; wounds; stammering.

Terminalia chebula { haritaki / harmaj } Nose-bleeding.

Thalictrum foliosum (tayman)—Wounds.

Thorn apple (dhaturo)—Pain in the stomach; guinea worms; pain in the vagina; piles; consumption; excessive menstruation.

Three-leaved chaste tree { nigod / nigadu

Tin (kathul)—

Tinospora cordifolia } amarsatva / galo { Tongue diseases; swelling; dysentery; gonorrhœa.

Treacle—Swelling; gonorrhœa; piles.

Trianthema crystallina (punarnava)—

Trianthema monogyne (vasith)—Delirium.

Trichosanthe cucumerina { katu- / patol / patol-beej } Wounds.

Troiling eclipta (bhangaro)—Hair dye; piles.

Turbeeth root	nasotar nisot shyman	Delirium; poisoning of rabid dog.
Turmeric	nisha rajmi	Itch; jaundice; pain in the stomach; guinea worms; swelling; leprosy; nose fistula; gonorrhœa; blood-poisoning; mauling by the tiger; wounds; scrofula.

Vejja Turkey (ativakh)—Diarrhœa.
Vitriol blue (morthuthu)—Itch; syphilis; piles; ulcers; tooth-ache; wounds; scrofula.
Vitriol green (hirakashi)—Piles.
Vraria picta (pidhavani)—Dysentery.

W

White clay (gopi chandan)—Ecthyma.
White sublimate (raskapur)—Ecthyma.
Winter cherries (asandh)—Tooth-ache; gonorrhœa; poison of serpent.
Witchania somnifera (asandh)—

Yellow orpiment (hadtal)—Itch; piles.

Zelory (kachoor)—

AN ADDITIONAL LIST OF INDIAN DRUGS, WOODS AND DYES WITH THEIR ENGLISH EQUIVALENTS

Abhul—Common juniper.
Adamvara—Common fig.
Afeen—Opium.
Agarch—Chaff flower.
Agaru—Eaglewood.
Ajmo—Apium involucratum.
Akola—Nutmeg—aleurites triloba, in reality two.
Akund—*See* arka.
Akurkaro—Indian fever.
Aloo—Caladium.
Aloo-ba-loo—Cherry.
Alu—*See* Batata.
Alwaine—Common cress.
Am—Mango.
Ambali—Common tamarind.
Ambar—Amber.
Ambli—Tamarind.
Amla—Shrubby phyllanthus.
Amlika—Emblic myrobalan-shrubby phyllanthus.
Amlika—Procumbent oxalis.
Amra—*See* am.
Amrita—*See* amla.
Amrool—*See* amlika.
Amulki—*See* amrita.
Anasphal—The capsule of the star-anise.
Anesun—Anise seed.
Anjana—Hardwickia binata.
Anjeer—Common fig.
Ananas—Common pineapple.
Aoon—Terminalia glabra.
Apamarga—*See* agarch.

Aparajita—Wing-leaved chitoria.
Arad—Small-fruited kidney bean.
Aralu—Indian ailanthus.
Arhuka—Two-coloured pigeon pea.
Arita—Emarquinated soap berry.
Arjuna—Terminalia arjuna.
Arka—Curled flowered calotropis.
Arkado—*See* arka.
Arunya—Common rice.
Ashratham—Arostigma religiosum.
Aswagandhi—Flegwose winter cherry.
Atasi—Common flax.
Atchi—Broad-leaved morinda.
Atees—Aconitum heteraphyllium.

B

Baboonee—Phual-Chamomile.
Babul—Gum Arabic tree.
Badami—Malay almond.
Badrang-buych—Common balm.
Bael—*See* shriphala.
Bagberanda—Angular-leaved physic nut.
Bahubami—Common marvel of Peru.
Bakla—Common kidney bean.
Bans—Common bamboo cane.
Bartung—Flea-wort.
Batata—Potato.
Bedana—Common quince.
Beejara-sala—*See* kaju.
Beendi—Eatable hibiscus, ochro.
Behura—Terminalia bellerica.
Bherlee-movra—Torn-leaved caryota.
Bhilaya—Marking nut.
Bhimb—Coccinia Indica.

Cariari—Superb gloriosa.
Chakso—Flour-leaved cursia.

Chalita—Large-flowered dellenia.
Chandana—True sandalwood.
Chandari—Winged pea.
Channa—Common gram ; common chick pea.
Chaunro—Chinese dolichos.
Chawl—Common rice.
Chilghaza—Pine nuts.
China narangi—Three-leaved triphasia.
Chitra—Plumbago rosea.
Choka—*See* chawl.
Choob-chinee—Chinese smilax.
Choroli—Buchanania latifolia.
Chosa—Garden poppy.
Chowlee—*See* Chaunro.
Chucuck-sawyeh—Arabian glass wort.
Chuko—Bladder dock.

Dadam—Pomegranate.
Dalchini—*See* davasita.
Damal-ook-wain—Resin ; dragon's blood.
Dantik—Purging croton.
Darchini—The leaf of the cinnamomum.
Dariya-ka-narel—*See* Narikel.
Davasita—Cinnamon (cinnamomum zeylanica).
Deodhan—Andrapon saccharatus.
Dhana—Indian wormwood.
Dhanaya—Coriander seeds.
Dharamputra—Virginian tobacco.
Dharu—Green-rooted turmeric.
Dhatura—Purple thorn apple.
Dhoondool-ghoora—Luffa pentadra.
Dhoop—Frankincense.
Doorla—Creeping cynodon.
Drakaha—Common grape.
Dudhi—Vegetable marrow.
Duk-nirbisi—The root pareira.
Durva—Creeping cynodon.

E

Erandi—Angular-leaved physic nut.
Erminakullie—Oleander-leaved cacalia.

F

Fudina—Tall red mint.
Ful—Garden bean.

G

Ganja—Hemp. (The Hashish of the Arabs comes from the tender tops of the plants after flowering.)
Ganjo—Common hemp.
Gardul—*See* Gila.
Garnikura—Hemp-leaved hibiscus.
Ghasul—*See* chubuck-ṣawyeh.
Ghundaha-bena—Lemon grass.
Gila—Entada pursætha.
Gokoru—Small caltrops.
Gokru—Turnip.
Googul—Indian bdellium.
Gooya-baboola—Sponge tree.
Gudar—*See* babul.
Gujar—The fœtid gum-resin-sarcocolla.
Guj-pipal—Officinal scindaspus.
Gul-hamax—Dentated dock.
Gulab—Cabbage rose.
Gulab-jam—Rose apple.
Gumbharee—Emelina arborea.
Gund—Narrow-leaved cordia.
Gundi—*See* gund.
Guraka—The nut of the medicinal cabbage tree.
Guvai—Cyamposis psoraloides.
Guvaka—Betel nut.

H

Halda—*See* Dharu.
Haleem—Common cress.
Hansraj—Maiden-hair fern.
Harenso—Common pea.
Hariphul—Long-leaved cicca.
Haritaka—Chebulic myrobalan.[1]
Harfarori—Long-leaved cicca.
Haridra—Long-rooted turmeric.
Haritika—Oval-leaved terminalia.
Hathagoon—Common cyclamen.
Hath-soda—*See* lakhmani.
Hathajuri—*See* hathagoon.
Heera-bol—Myrrh.
Heerda—*See* Haritika.
Hilyoon—Common asparagus.
Hinduba—Wild succory.
Hing—Asafœtida.
Hoober—*See* Pudma.
Hubul-Ghur-Laurus Nobilis—the true laurel of the poet and student—their crown was of sweet bay in berry, from which comes "bachelor" (bacca laureatus).
Huldi—*See* harida.
Huluka—Nymphæa lotus.
Hunfarori—*See* hariphul.

I

Imborel—Indian madan.
Indravaruni—The bitter cucumber-colocynth.
Irkamula—Indian birthwort.
Irsa—Orris root.
Ispagul—Spogel seed.
Ishwara—*See* irkamula.

[1] *See* first index. These are arranged in six classes:
(1) Helilah-zireh—The fruit dried when just formed, and the size of a cumin seed (zira).
(2) Helileh-jawi—The fruit dried when the size of a barley-corn (java).
(3) Helileh-zengi—The fruit dried when the size of a raisin, and black like a negro (zengi).
(4) Helileh-chini—The fruit dried when the size of green gram (chini).
(5) Helileh-asfer—The fruit near maturity and yellow (asfer).
(6) Helileh-kabuli—The fruit at full maturity.

J

Jambul—Syzygium jambolanum.
Jangli-piaz—Urginea Indica.
Jarasaya—Cherry.
Jayfal—*See* Akola.
Jeera—Cumin seeds.
Jetamasi—Spikenard.
Jethimadh—Common liquorice.
Jivanputra—Putranjiva roxburgh—Wild olives.
Jowari-joar-juwar—Indian millet.
Jungli-badam—Broad-leaved terminalia.
Juwashur—The gum-resin, opponax.
Jydaroomee—*See* Damal-ook-wain.

K

Kachura—Broad-leaved turmeric.
Kadali—Common plantain.
Kaju—Common cashew.
Kakadi—Cucumis utiliosimus.
Kakmari—The berry of the cocculas Indicus.
Kalajeera—Small fennel flower.
Kala-moong—Hairy padded kidney bean.
Kalikekar—Gum Arabic tree.
Kalitulshi—Common sweet basil.
Kalu—Common peach.
Kalumbi—White Malabar nightshade.
Kalyana—Greater galangal.
Kam-aloo-wing—Stalked yam.
Kamarunga—*See* bilimba.
Kamla—Lotus.
Kaner—Sweet-scented oleander.
Kanjir—Garden artichoke.
Kantal—Artocarpus integrifolia.
Kapitha—Indian elephant apple.
Karanda—*See* Krishnapak-phul.
Karela—Hairy momordica.
Karelo-jangro—Balsam apple.
Kariyatu—Chiretta.
Karpasa—Common cotton.

Karpura—Camphor.
Kartoli—Momordica dioica.
Karu-karrinda—Bulb-bearing yam.
Kasha—The culm of saccharum.
Katuroum—Christmas rose (the root black hellebore).
Kavach—*See* kowchanj.
Kawa—Arabian coffee.
Kayaput-ki-tel—Cajput oil.
Keerakankari—Common cucumber.
Kela—Common plantain.
Kemboo—Showy costus.
Kemooka—*See* kemboo.
Kepoor-amber—
Keraji—Celery.
Keri—Common mango.
Keril—Capparis aphylla.
Keshoor—*See* punnaga.
Keshur—Dyers rottlera.
Ketuka—Green-spined screw pine.
Keysur—Saffron crocus.
Khadira, medical acacia—Catechu.
Khajur-khajuri—Wood date palm.
Kheeri—Obtuse-leaved mimusops.
Khernoob-shamee—Carot tree.
Khijdi—*See* gooya-baboole.
Khorasani ajwan—Common henbane.
Khurjiooree—Date.
Kidamari—Bractrated birth wort.
Kobi—Cabbage.
Kokum—Garcinia purpurea.
Koharoo—Pumpkin.
Koli—Blunt-leaved zizypus.
Koolti—Two-flowered dolichos.
Koonch—Jamaica wild liquorice.
Koondur rumi—Mastic tree.
Korudoosha—Punctured paspalum.
Kowchanj—Indian cowhage.
Kowut—Common sapota.
Krishnapak-phul—Jasmine-flowered cassia.
Kubel—Sweet calamus.
Kuchandana—Yellow-flowered adenathera.

Kuchila—Poison, nut.
Kuchwee—Egyptian arum.
Kudsumba—The pod of canavalia virosa.
Kudsumber—Salre-padded canavalia.
Kuknuj—Stocks.
Kundah—*See* sooran.
Kundel—The gum resin, sagapenum.
Kunkuma—Gardenia lucida, gardenia gummifera.
Kurmah—Date.
Kursah—Parsley.
Kurwa-badam—Bitter almonds.
Kusambha—Officinal carthamus.
Kusha—Poa cynosuroides.
Kuskus—Andropogon muricatus.
Krishna-jiraka—The black cumin of scripture.
Kussoos—*See* lublub.
Kust—Costus.
Kusumbha—Safflower.
Kutaka—Clearing nut.
Kuveraka—Indian bastard cedar.

Lohoree-hoormul—Syrian rue.
Lakhami—Officinal mandrake.
Lakoocha—Artocapus lakoocha.
Lal behmen—Bloody vemed sage.
Lal jamphul—Red guava.
Lang—Chickling vetch.
Lanka-sij—Indian tree spurge.
Lavinga—Clove.
Litchi—Nephelium litchi.
Loba—*See* bakla.
Lobani-ood—Benzoin.
Loonia—Small purslani.
Lublub—Common ivy.

M

Mag—Rajed kidney bean.
Maidalakdi—Tetranthera roxburghu.

Majuphal—Nut galls.
Malaka-jambu—Malay apple.
Mandra—Indian coral tree.
Manpul—*See* majuphul.
Maricha—Black pepper.
Marchaina—Three-leaved yam.
Marwa—Sweet marjorum.
Masoor—Lentil.
Mazuyoon—Merzereon or spurge olive.
Meeshmee teeta—Coptis teeta.
Meetha kamarunga—Carambola.
Meih-seela—Rose malloes ; liquadambar of the sweet gum tree.
Menali viceray—Trailing gisekia.
Mendi—Henna plant.
Mesta—Roselle.
Methi—Fennugreek.
Mokka—Common Indian corn.
Mon-aloo—Prickly stemmed yam.
Mooluka—Common radish.
Moong—*See* mag.
Moong-phuli—American earth nut.
Movra—*See* madhuka.
Mukshun-shim—*See* kudsumber.
Muli—*See* mooluka.
Mulu vangay—Prickly birdelia.
Mungeestun—Common mangosteen.
Murha—Thick spiked eleusine.
Mushabir—Aloes.
Musli—The voot stalk.
Mutasi—*See* atasi.

N

Nagdan—Poison bulb cumin.
Nagdown—Common asparagus.
Nagdowna—Mug wort.
Nagkeshar—Mesna ferrea.
Nagmootha—The root of cyperus pertenius.
Nagputra—Turbith.
Nakchinkni—Sneez wort.
Naranga—Sweet orange.

Narel—*See* narikel.
Narikel—Common coconut.
Nella-neem—Ash-leaved bean tree.
Nella-shama—Panicum meliare.
Nilkulmi—Morning glory.
Nil-padma—Star-flowered water lily.
Nimba—*See* neem.
Nimbuka—Bergamot citrus.
Nirbishi—Antidote to bish-dephinium pancifloram.
Nirghoondi—*See* Sindhuva.

O

Oka-mundel—The fruit of the down palm ; gingerbread tree.
Ood—Benzoin.
Ood-i-balasun—Balsam.
Oshak—Eastern giant fennel.

P

Padel—Trumpet flower.
Padma—Lotus, Egyptian.
Padri—*See* padel.
Palandu—Common onion.
Palas—Downy-branched butea.
Paluk—Common spinach.
Panawla—Esculint flacourtia.
Pan—Betel pepper.
Pangri—Indian coral tree.
Papaya—Common papau.
Papeeta—St. Ignatius bean.
Parnasa—Purple-stalked basil (sacred to Vishnu).
Patrabanga—*See* kidamari.
Peeas—Common onion.
Peeta—Long-rooted turmeric.
Pharsi—Panicled dalbergia.
Phulsha—Asiatic grewia.
Pippla—Arostigma religiosum.
Pippali—Long pepper.

Pista—Pistachio.
Poodina—Tall red-mint.
Pudma—Common juniper.
Pulsha—Asiatic grewia.
Punaga—Dyers rottlera.
Pundeetuka—Prickly vanguierria.
Punnaga—The powder on the capsule, kamala.
Purava—Common snake gourd.
Puti-karanja—Oval-leaved nicker tree.
Putranga—Red wood.
Putta—Heart-leaved corchorus.
Putu-toddy—The fermented sap of the palmyra.

R

Rai—Thick spiked eleusine.
Rajani-gandha—Common tuberose.
Rajika—Species of mustard.
Rajputako—*See* kuknuj.
Rakta-chitraka—Rose-coloured lead wort.
Ramphul—Netted custard apple.
Ram-sita—Netted custard apple.
Rasala—Sugar cane.
Ratakodol—Common yam.
Rata-nil-nakuta—Jamaica bastard verbani.
Rewund chini—Officinal rhubarb.
Ringana—*See* vegan.
Rohuna—Febrifuge soymida.
Rudraksha—Elacocarpus ganitrus.
Ruriya—Large-flowered dellenia.

S

Safaid jamphal—White guava.
Safaid musli—Murdannia scapifolia.
Safaid behmen—Saw-leaved centaury.
Safrajan—*See* seba.
Saigut—*See* sigru.
Sakar-kor—Melon pumpkin.

Salbia—Garden sage.
Salep-musree—The root, oriental salef (orchid class).
Salim-musree—*See* salep musree.
Sama-samo—Panicum frumentaceum.
Samundra-phul—Barringtonia acutangula.
Sanji—*See* Bahubami.
Sarasav—Mustard.
Sarass—Common cypress.
Saurij—Anise-seed.
Shahbullol—Barbarry oak.
Shalgram—Turnip.
Sharkara-kand—Sweet potato.
Shatavari—Roof of linear-leaved asparagus.
Sheba—Apple.
Sheloo—Cordia latifolia.
Sheradi—*See* Rasala.
Shetura—Mulberry.
Shirkhist—Mana.
Shriphala—Thorny Bengal quince.
Shyamaka—*See* Samo.
Sigru—Smooth horseradish tree.
Sillarus—The balsam.
Sindica—*See* timbin.
Sindhuva—Three-leaved chaste tree.
Sita-phul—*See* Ram-sita, Ramphul.
Sobhayan—Smooth horseradish tree.
Soma—Twisting sarcostemnia.
Somalata—*See* soma.
Sooran—Campanulate amorphophallus.
Sopari—Betel nut.
Spar—Garden thyme.
Sudab—Narrow-leaved rose.
Sugandha-maricha—Cubeb.
Sukhdarsoon—*See* nagdan.
Sug-ungoor—Deadly nightshade.
Sulk—Common beet.
Suparas havaka—Poplar-leaved hibiscus.
Sursan—*See* rajika.
Sukhmuniya—Scammony.
Sunamukhi—Senna.
Supari—*See* guraka.

Suru—Common cypress.
Suva—Dill seeds.
Suvanuka—Cassia.
Swadu-kuntuka—*See* panawla.

T

Tadulia—Eatable amaranth.
Taj—Cassia lignes—The bark of the cinnamomum cassia. (*See* dalchini.)
Tal—*See* putu-toddy.
Tamaku—Virginian tobacco.
Tamal-patra—The leaf of the cinnamomum tamala.
Tamrakoota—*See* Tamaku.
Tapuria—Eatable winter cherry.
Tar—Palmyra.
Tarbuch—Water melon.
Tejbul—Indian tooth-ache tree.
Thoono—Common yew.
Timbin—Diospyros glutinosa.
Toom—Wing-leaved garuga.
Trivínta—*See* nagputra.
Tucker—Asarabica.
Tulisha—Many-spined flacourtia.
Tuna—*See* kuveraka.
Turi—Acute-angled cucumber.
Tuvar—Two-coloured pigeon pea.

U

Umbir—Amber.
Urtenysa—*See* hathagoori.
Ustakhudus—French lavender.
Ustarak—Officinal storax.

Vacha—Sweet-flag.
Vahirsee—*See* kartoli
Vaj—Sweet-flag.

Valpapadi—Black-seeded dolichos.

Vana-adrukam—Downy-leaved ginger.

Vanraj—Small flowered mountain ebony. Acacia concinna—the seeds of this plant are used as weights: Gunja, gr. 15/10 apothecary's weight. The seeds are also called in medicine ratika, and ten ratis (ratikas) are equal to one "mashaka" and eight "mashaka" one tola.

Vansha—Common bamboo cane.

Vas—*See* vansha.

Variyali—Fennel seed, aniseed.

Vatana—Common pea.

Vavading—Embelia ribes, the fruit.

Vegan—Egg plant.

Vijya—*See* bhang and ganja.

Vilati mendi—Common myrtle.

Vilayati gas—Lucerne.

Vilva-ham—Holy garlic pear.

Vimbika—*See* bhimb.

Viskamandala—*See* nagadan.

Vrihih-heda—Millet.

W

Walvangi—Love apple, tomato.

Y

Yava—Winter barley.

Z

Zajnee—The berry of sweet bay.

Zeerah—Black carraway seed.

Zerawund-mooderaj—*See* zerawund, tuweel.

Zerawund-tuweel—Long-rooted birth wort.

Zoofæ teabus—Common hyssop.